Palgrave Studies in Public Health Policy Research

Public health has increasingly cast the net wider. The field has moved on from a hygiene perspective and infectious and occupational disease base (where it was born in the 19th century) to a concern for unhealthy lifestyles post-WWII, and more recently to the uneven distribution of health and its (re)sources. It is of course interesting that these 'paradigms' in many places around the world live right next to each other. Hygiene, lifestyles, and health equity form the complex (indeed, wicked) policy agendas for health and social/sustainable development. All of these, it is now recognized, are part of the 'social determinants of health'.

The broad new public health agenda, with its multitude of competing issues, professions, and perspectives requires a much more sophisticated understanding of government and the policy process. In effect, there is a growing recognition of the extent to which the public health community writ large needs to better understand government and move beyond what has traditionally been a certain naiveté about politics and the process of policy making. Public health scholars and practitioners have embraced this need to understand, and influence, how governments at all levels make policy choices and decisions. Political scientists and international relations scholars and practitioners are engaging in the growing public health agenda as it forms an interesting expanse of glocal policy development and implementation.

Broader, more detailed, and more profound scholarship is required at the interface between health and political science. This series will thus be a powerful tool to build bridges between political science, international relations and public health. It will showcase the potential of rigorous political and international relations science for better understanding public health issues. It will also support the public health professional with a new theoretical and methodological toolbox. The series will include monographs (both conventional and shorter Pivots) and collections that appeal to three audiences: scholars of public health, public health practitioners, and members of the political science community with an interest in public health policy and politics.

More information about this series at
http://www.palgrave.com/gp/series/15414

Benjamin Hawkins · Chris Holden ·
Sophie Mackinder

The Battle for Standardised Cigarette Packaging in Europe

Multi-Level Governance, Policy Transfer and the Integrated Strategy of the Global Tobacco Industry

palgrave
macmillan

Benjamin Hawkins
London School of Hygiene
& Tropical Medicine
London, UK

Chris Holden
University of York
York, North Yorkshire, UK

Sophie Mackinder
Social Policy and Social Work
University of York
York, North Yorkshire, UK

Palgrave Studies in Public Health Policy Research
ISBN 978-3-030-31033-2 ISBN 978-3-030-31034-9 (eBook)
https://doi.org/10.1007/978-3-030-31034-9

Cover credit: PjrTravel/Alamy Stock Photo

This Palgrave Pivot imprint is published by the registered company Springer Nature Switzerland AG
The registered company address is: Gewerbestrasse 11, 6330 Cham, Switzerland

For Sharon and Chris Hawkins

Acknowledgements

We would like to thank the National Cancer Institute, US National Institutes of Health, for funding the research project from which this book draws (Grant Number R01-CA091021). In addition, we would like to thank Professor Kelley Lee and Dr. Ross MacKenzie for their advice on the development of the book and comments on aspects of the text. We would also like to thank Jennifer Fang and the administrative teams at Simon Fraser University, the London School of Hygiene and Tropical Medicine and the University of York for all their work in supporting this research. Finally, we would like to thank all those who responded to requests for interviews or other information during the course of our research.

Contents

About the Authors

Dr. Benjamin Hawkins is Assistant Professor in the Department of Global Health and Development at the London School of Hygiene and Tropical Medicine. His research focuses principally on the role of corporate actors on alcohol and tobacco regulation. In addition, he has published work on European integration, multi-level governance, international trade and political economy approaches to health policy.

Dr. Chris Holden is Reader in International Social Policy at the University of York, UK. He has published widely on the relationships between the global economy, transnational corporations and health and social policy. He has been a member of the Executive Committee of the UK Social Policy Association, the Editorial Board of the *Journal of Social Policy* and the International Advisory Board of *Global Social Policy*.

Dr. Sophie Mackinder is Associate Lecturer in International Development and Global Social Policy at the University of York, UK. She recently completed her Ph.D. on social protection, fragile states and the World Bank.

Abbreviations

ALDE	Alliance of Liberals and Democrats for Europe
ASH	Action on Smoking and Health
BAT	British American Tobacco
BIT	Bilateral Investment Treaty
CJEU	Court of Justice of the EU
CNTC	Chinese National Tobacco Corporation
CRUK	Cancer Research UK
DG	Directorate General
DSB	Dispute Settlement Body
ECL	Association of European Cancer Leagues
EEC	European Economic Community
ENVI	Committee on Environment, Public Health and Food Safety
EP	European Parliament
EPP	European People's Party
EU	European Union
FCTC	Framework Convention on Tobacco Control
FDI	Foreign Direct Investment
FOI	Freedom of Information
IBEC	Irish Business & Employers Confederation
ICS	Irish Cancer Society
IHF	Irish Heart Foundation
IMF	International Monetary Fund
IP	Intellectual Property
ISDS	Investor-State Dispute Settlement
ITMAC	Irish Tobacco Manufacturers Association
JTI	Japan Tobacco International

JURI	Committee on Legal Affairs
LMIC	Low and Middle-Income Countries
MEP	Member of the European Parliament
MLG	Multi-Level Governance
NGO	Non-Governmental Organisation
NPM	New Public Management
PM	Philip Morris
PMI	Philip Morris International
PR	Public Relations
QMV	Qualified Majority Voting
S&D	Progressive Alliance of Socialists and Democrats
SFP	Smoke Free Partnership
SP	Standardised Packaging
TD	Teachta Dála
TEU	Treaty on European Union
TFEU	Treaty on the Functioning of the EU
TPD	Tobacco Products Directive
TTC	Transnational Tobacco Company
UK	United Kingdom
UKIP	UK Independence Party
UN	United Nations
US	United States
WHO	World Health Organization
WTO	World Trade Organization

CHAPTER 1

Introduction

Abstract This book analyses the battle for standardised cigarette packaging ('plain packaging') in Europe, drawing on the concepts of multi-level governance and policy transfer. This chapter provides the global context of the policy processes examined in the book and sets out the book's aims and structure. It explains the importance of branding and pack design to transnational tobacco companies (TTCs), and details the emergence of related tobacco-control measures outside of Europe. In particular, it focuses on the introduction of standardised packaging in Australia. It then describes TTC political strategies in opposing such measures, via trade litigation and other methods. The chapter also sets out the research methods used to collect and analyse the empirical data used in the book.

Keywords Introduction · Methods · Standardised tobacco packaging · Plain packaging · Transnational tobacco companies

The global cigarette industry is dominated by a small number of transnational tobacco companies (TTCs). Outside of China, in which over 90% of the market is overseen by the state-controlled Chinese National Tobacco Corporation (CNTC), these corporations operate as oligopolies, dominating national cigarette markets, and enjoying significant ability to segment

B. Hawkins et al., *The Battle for Standardised Cigarette Packaging in Europe*, Palgrave Studies in Public Health Policy Research,
https://doi.org/10.1007/978-3-030-31034-9_1

markets and control price points (CFTFKs 2018). In addition, TTCs pursue sophisticated marketing strategies, which have been shown to drive sales, consumption and harms when they enter new markets (Hafez and Ling 2005; Hawkins et al. 2016, 2018). Given the high level of fungibility between manufactured cigarettes—which in the words of tobacco industry whistle-blower Jeffrey Wigand are simply 'nicotine delivery' devices—differentiation between products depends almost exclusively on branding activity (Wigand 1996). The importance of branding and marketing to the cigarette industry is evident not only in the extensive history of industry advertising and celebrity endorsements over decades, but also in the vehemence with which they have opposed attempts to curtail their ability to advertise or promote their wares by national governments, at the European Union (EU) level and within the context of the World Health Organization's (WHO) Framework Convention on Tobacco Control (FCTC) (Savell et al. 2014). Moreover, restrictions on marketing are correlated with reductions in smoking prevalence across the globe (WHO 2008), underlining the crucial role that marketing plays in recruiting and retaining smokers, with deleterious effects on public health. In many settings, including much of Europe, bans on television, cinema, magazine and billboard advertising meant the cigarette pack itself became one of the last available conduits available to tobacco producers to market their products. Consequently, the removal of colour branding and the introduction of standardised packaging (SP) for cigarettes, first in Australia and subsequently in several EU member states, posed a key strategic threat to industry actors, which they vehemently opposed. This book builds on previous studies of the battle for SP in Australia and elsewhere (Chapman and Freeman 2014; Jarman 2015) to examine how SP came onto the policy agenda in Europe, how its adoption was prevented by the industry at the EU level, and how individual member states subsequently succeeded in introducing it in the face of fierce industry opposition.

Transnational Tobacco Companies and Political Strategy

TTCs are formidable political actors. A now extensive literature—which has drawn on internal company documents released into the public domain from the mid-1990s—has documented the extent of their efforts to resist regulation and shape the policy environments in which they operate (Gilmore 2012; Hurt et al. 2009; Holden and Lee 2009; Smith et al. 2013;

Savell et al. 2014). Strategies employed by the industry include extensive political lobbying and financial contributions to political candidates and parties; the funding of 'scientific' research, and the formation of front groups to cast doubt on scientific evidence that identifies the harms associated with smoking and the effectiveness of policy interventions designed to reduce consumption (Bero 2005; Hurt et al. 2009; Savell et al. 2014; Smith et al. 2013; Brandt 2012). As information about the tactics of the industry entered the public consciousness and concerns about the conflicts of interest involved in TTCs' engagement with health policy-makers began to solidify, TTCs began to be marginalised from the policy process in many contexts. This culminated with the inclusion of Article 5.3 in the FCTC, which commits signatories to take pro-active measures to guard against the influence of the tobacco industry over policy (WHO 2003). The normative force derived from such an explicit recognition of the issues surrounding the tobacco industry within a global treaty has meant direct and overt engagement with tobacco industry actors is politically controversial in many settings, although implementation of Article 5.3 remains piecemeal, and political access away from the public spotlight is still possible (Fooks et al. 2017; Hawkins and Holden 2018). Industry influence remains extensive, particularly in strategically important low and middle-income country (LMIC) settings, and TTC strategies have evolved to take account of these changed political realities.

As their ability to engage decision-makers has been curtailed in many settings, TTCs have developed both more covert and more confrontational strategies to achieve their political objectives. This has involved, for example, the use of cross-industry trade bodies to represent their interests within the context of broader policy negotiations such as international trade agreements (Hawkins et al. 2018). Where specific tobacco industry interests are at stake, such as during the revision to the EU Tobacco Products Directive (TPD) examined below, or with the introduction of SP in Australia, industry actors have begun to use legal challenges in an attempt to prevent, or at least amend and/or delay, measures designed to reduce smoking and thus the consumption of their products (Hawkins and Holden 2016; Holden and Hawkins 2017). These challenges may be brought under international trade law via the World Trade Organization (WTO), EU single-market law or, more recently, under the auspices of bilateral investment treaties (BITs). The latter often include investor-state dispute settlement (ISDS) mechanisms, which offer private companies the ability to take direct legal action against state governments which they claim have infringed their rights as investors (Hawkins and Holden 2016).

In parallel with the partial political marginalisation of the tobacco industry, the ability of TTCs to market their products has also been increasingly restricted (see Henriksen 2012), in line with best-practice guidelines set out in the FCTC (WHO 2013). Marketing restrictions have led TTCs to become increasingly reliant on pricing differentiation and market segmentation to attract and retain smokers (Gilmore et al. 2010). As with Article 5.3 compliance, the degree to which tobacco marketing is restricted varies greatly from region to region and country to country. Even in Europe, a region with one of the most advanced bodies of tobacco-control regulation globally, and in which much tobacco policy, at least for EU member states (and those within the broader regulatory orbit of the EU), is adopted collectively at the European level, there is significant variation in the ability of tobacco companies to market their products (Bertollini et al. 2016). For example, most forms of marketing such as television and magazine advertising are banned in the EU under the 1998 Tobacco Advertising Directive (98/43/EC) (see Neuman et al. 2002). Yet other media fall under the national, rather than the EU, remit. In Germany, billboard advertising and cinema advertising, which do not have cross-border effects and thus fall outside the remit of EU law, are still permitted, while in countries such as the UK and Ireland these have been eliminated. Given the decreasing range of potential outlets for industry marketing activities, the cigarette pack itself has taken on increasing significance for the industry as one of the few remaining ways in which producers can communicate with existing and potential customers in many settings. Consequently, they have used all available resources to defend their ability to brand packaging in the face of increasingly large warning labels (which both highlight the harms of smoking and reduce the space available for branding) and attempts to introduce 'plain' or standardised packaging, in which all differentiation in packaging between brands in terms of shape, size, form and colour, is removed. We follow the lead of health NGOs interviewed during the course of our study in using the term 'standardised packaging' (SP) rather than 'plain packaging' in the analysis below. Policy advocates favoured this language in order to avoid the misconception during the development of the policy that it would lead to the removal of graphic and written health warnings as well as industry logos and colour palates.

TTC Challenges to Tobacco Packaging Measures

The strategy of using international trade law to challenge tobacco product packaging measures was first evident in response to attempts by the Uruguayan government to introduce larger graphic warning labels on cigarette packets and further restrictions on the branding and descriptions of cigarettes (Jarman 2015; Hawkins and Holden 2016). Action was taken by Philip Morris International under the Switzerland–Uruguay BIT to oppose these measures, with the arbitration panel finding in favour of Uruguay, although not until the country had incurred significant material and non-material costs which were only partially compensated by the final judgement (Olivet and Villareal 2016). The vehemence of the industry response to developments in Uruguay appears to have been motivated not by domestic concerns, in a small country with limited TTC penetration, but by TTCs' desire to prevent ***policy contagion*** to larger, strategically important markets and to test the ability to prevent such measures using BITs. Success would deter other countries tempted to follow suit, by making clear TTCs' intention to oppose such measures and the costs involved in fighting their claims. This is in keeping with previous work on the alcohol industry—which has been shown to pursue a closely related political ***modus operandi*** to the tobacco industry—which found that corporate activities to oppose policy decisions taken in one jurisdiction are often driven by political imperatives not in that jurisdiction, but by those elsewhere (i.e. in key strategic markets) or by broader, global, strategic imperatives (Holden and Hawkins 2013; Hawkins et al. 2018).

The decision by the Australian government to introduce SP for cigarettes in 2012 gave rise to a further wave of litigation under WTO rules and under the ISDS mechanisms of the Australia–Hong Kong BIT (Jarman 2015; Chapman and Freeman 2014; Hawkins and Holden 2016; Hawkins et al. 2018). The objectives for the industry were similar to those in the Uruguay case, but related directly to SP. In challenging Australia, the TTCs' aim was not only to defend sales in this declining market, but to prevent further policy contagion to other markets and to create a 'chilling' effect on other states considering similar action. The instigation of proceedings under WTO law by five WTO member states funded by the tobacco industry potentially allowed the plaintiffs to create a precedent that such policies violate international trade law, and thus to stymie its potential introduction in all WTO member states at a single stroke. The Australian government won its case before the WTO, with the dispute settlement panel circulating its case report to parties on 28 June 2018 and the Dispute Settlement Body (DSB), adopting the report at its meeting on 27 August 2018. On 19 July 2018, one of the plaintiff countries, Honduras, announced its intention to appeal the decision to the WTO's Appellate Body and, at the time of writing, the final outcome of this process remains to be determined. The case brought under the Australia–Hong Kong BIT was resolved in favour of Australia also, but on technical grounds related to the timing of the transfer of ownership of Philip Morris' Australian holding company to its Hong Kong-based subsidiary, which occurred after the announcement of Australia's SP measures, thus rendering the claim inadmissible under the BIT. However, the substantive point of law remains to be tested and, as BITs vary both in their content and interpretation by disputes panels, countries party to BITs with ISDS mechanisms that seek to introduce SP remain vulnerable to challenges under those agreements.

Policy Transfer: From Australia to Europe

Following the introduction of SP in Australia, the policy came onto the agenda in other policy settings, including at the EU level in the context of the 2014 revision of the TPD and within several EU member states. This represented precisely the kind of 'policy contagion' that the TTCs had feared, and which they had sought to avoid through the various legal challenges against Australia. Despite extensive regulation of the sale and use of their products and declining rates of consumption, Europe remains a key market for TTCs, accounting for significant sales volumes and profits. The introduction of SP in this context, alongside existing marketing restrictions, would thus be highly problematic for the tobacco industry. The powerful supranational legal instruments at the disposal of the EU—which it has used previously to enact significant tobacco control measures (Hervey 2001; McKee et al. 2010)—would mean that policies adopted at the EU level would be implemented at a single stroke in twenty-eight member states. Consequently, the potential adoption of SP within the TPD posed a significant threat to industry interests across a key strategic region.

As with challenges under WTO law, pursuing opposition to policies such as SP at the supranational level via the EU offers industry actors a parsimonious approach for preventing policy developments across multiple policy settings. However, where collective action at the EU level is prevented, member states are free to pursue policies at the national level, unless they are ruled to be incompatible with EU law by the Court of Justice of the

EU (CJEU). Thus, once proposals to implement SP at the European level were dropped from the proposed TPD (see Chapter 3; Peeters et al. 2015), preventing SP in whichever member state moved first was of the highest strategic importance to the industry. Adoption of such measures by any individual member state was a key priority to avoid because of the propensity for policy ideas to spread rapidly between member states once a new area of regulation is implemented in one. The close political and economic alignment between EU member states, and the existence of highly developed trans-European political, expert and NGO networks which facilitate this, provides an ideal context for such policy transfer or 'policy contagion'.

The policy processes on SP in Ireland and the UK were closely connected and developed in parallel. Ireland became the first country in the EU to enact legislation to introduce SP, with the Public Health (Standardised Packaging of Tobacco) Act 2015 signed into law by President Michael D. Higgins on 10 May 2015, a day before Members of Parliament voted to adopt similar measures in the UK. However, following delays in implementation in Ireland, the measures were introduced first in the UK. All cigarettes produced in the UK from 20 May 2016 had to be in SP, with a 12-month grace period to allow the sale of branded packs brought to market before this date. SP came into effect in Ireland on 30 September 2017 with a similar 12 month 'wash through' period for old branded stock. In adopting SP, Ireland continued its position at the cutting edge of tobacco-control policy in Europe, established in the early 2000s with its leadership on the introduction of the smoking ban in enclosed spaces. Given the commitment of the Irish government to SP, Ireland emerged as a key battleground for the tobacco industry in its campaign to prevent SP in Europe and the restrictions this would place on its ability to brand and market its products. The adoption of SP in Ireland and the UK was followed by the passage of similar measures in other member states, including France and Hungary.

As well as the development of SP, TTCs faced further challenges to their ability to brand and market their products in the EU in the form of the TPD which, despite the abandonment of SP measures, contained proposals to increase significantly the size and format of warning labels, whilst placing restrictions on the shape, size and minimum content of cigarette packs. The development of SP in member states must, therefore, be seen within the wider policy-making context of the EU's system of multi-level governance.

The Aims of This Book

This book seeks to build on the literature on the political strategies of the tobacco industry, as well as the role of tobacco-control advocates in supporting the development of evidence-based policy, by documenting the development of SP proposals in Europe. We do this through engagement with key concepts from political science: *multi-level governance* and *policy transfer*. In doing so, we also aim to make a contribution to the theoretical literature on policy transfer, particularly in relation to the role of non-state actors. Our previous work has demonstrated that TTCs have pursued highly coordinated, multi-level and multi-dimensional strategies to oppose new packaging and labelling requirements across various political settings (Hawkins et al. 2018). In addition, previous studies have identified the importance of international tobacco-control NGO networks in the successful development of tobacco-control policy and its spread across the globe (Gneiting and Schmitz 2016; Weishaar et al. 2016). Policy transfer and knowledge exchange between tobacco-control advocates is a crucial dimension of how SP came onto the agenda and was successfully implemented in Ireland, and how it spread to other member states.

Whilst much has been written about the battle to introduce SP in Australia, much less attention has been paid to TTC efforts to prevent 'policy contagion' in those countries which announced they would follow suit (Chapman and Freeman 2014; Voon et al. 2014; Jarman 2015). In other words, there have been only limited efforts to date to place the landmark developments in Australia, both in terms of the policy innovation of SP and the particular response of the tobacco industry to this, in a global context or to understand this in terms of policy transfer. Policy debates and industry political strategies, we argue, are highly interconnected, particularly in the context of such a highly concentrated, oligopolistic, global industry as tobacco. We focus on Europe in part because it was governments in this part of the world which most quickly followed Australia's lead. However, the process of European integration, and the concurrent moves by national governments to enact SP alongside the negotiations surrounding the EU TPD, make this a highly fertile terrain for investigating industry strategy simultaneously at different levels of governance and in different decision-making forums. In so doing, we aim to contribute to the literature on multi-level governance and policy transfer, and address the gap in the latter literature regarding the role of corporate actors in policy transfer processes.

In the following chapters, we examine the development of the TPD and the subsequent SP debates in Ireland. The focus on Ireland, versus larger member states, reflects not only the political leadership shown by the Irish government on tobacco control, but also the crucial role played by the Irish government in the passage of the TPD during its presidency of the Council of the European Union ('the Council') in the first semester of 2013. This allows us to explore the mutual imbrication of national and EU-level political processes and the extent to which TTCs used political strategies at each level to influence those at the other. Crucially also for this book, the focus on the TTC response to SP in Ireland—a small member state of around four million people with a rapidly declining cigarette market and extensive existing tobacco-control policies in place—highlights the global significance of national policy debates. As with the Uruguay dispute cited above, we argue that the vehemence of the TTCs' response to Ireland's SP proposals must be explained not in terms of the economic importance of that market, but in terms of the role it plays in a global campaign to prevent branding and labelling restrictions. It was designed to prevent policy 'contagion' initially to, and subsequently throughout, the EU and act as a deterrent to governments elsewhere considering the introduction of such policies. However, the close geographical and political ties between Ireland and the United Kingdom (UK), and the concurrent development of SP legislation there, meant that policy developments in the UK were also of relevance to the SP debate in Ireland, and will be discussed in this context. Finally, we discuss the role of Australia in the Irish SP debates, not just as a policy entrepreneur, but as a policy facilitator through the close engagement of tobacco-control advocates in each context via transnational advocacy networks. This allowed Irish NGOs to learn from the example and experience of their Australian colleagues in understanding and responding to tobacco industry strategies to oppose SP.

Methodology

The analysis presented in this volume is drawn from a wider study of the tobacco industry's evolving political strategy in the context of globalisation. It is informed by, and makes a contribution to, key concepts derived from political science, principally policy transfer and multi-level governance, which are discussed in detail in the following chapter. In keeping with this, we employ qualitative research methods, which allow us to trace the evolution of tobacco packaging policy at the EU level and in key member states, the interconnections between these, and their relationship with global tobacco-control developments. In keeping with the principle of triangulation, we analyse both documentary and interview sources to examine these policy developments.

Case selection was purposive, and the decision to focus on Ireland, versus other EU member states, reflects the political leadership of Ireland on tobacco control in the region, both at the EU level via its Presidency of the Council at a key stage in the conclusion of the TPD, and through its political commitment to introducing SP at the national level. Whilst the SP policy process in the UK developed largely in parallel with that of Ireland—with the UK becoming the second EU member state to pass such legislation just days after its neighbour—there was far less clear political commitment to the development of the policy in Westminster compared to Dublin. Having committed themselves to introducing SP following a public consultation in 2012, the UK's coalition government equivocated on the issue, omitting it from the 2013 Queen's Speech and announcing in July 2013 that they would 'wait and see' how the policy played out in Australia, before bringing forward legislation. Following widespread criticism from the public health community, the UK government reversed its decision. Meanwhile, the Irish government announced its firm intention to become the first European country to introduce SP in May 2013. Consequently, we view Ireland as the political leader in Europe on this issue and the key focus of our analysis at the national level. Yet, as in so many other areas, the history of Irish tobacco-control policy is greatly influenced by developments in the UK. As such, we examine the interconnections between policy debates and key policy actors in both settings, but do so from the perspective of Ireland as the key regional policy entrepreneur.

Documentary analysis was undertaken in the context of a wider study of the development of tobacco packaging policy and tobacco industry counter-strategy globally, including the UK and Ireland (see Hawkins et al. 2018). Documents relating to these processes were retrieved by SM from online searches relating to policy debates on tobacco products packaging in relevant jurisdictions and industry responses to policy requirements, including documents relating to litigation in domestic courts and trade and investment disputes in bilateral and regional forums and the WTO. Internet searches were conducted initially using keywords relating to the relevant tobacco packaging legislation in each jurisdiction. Thereafter a 'snowballing' search technique was used to follow up sources and key phrases cited in the documents initially retrieved. Documents originating from relevant sources such as government departments, courts, international agencies, tobacco companies or allied organisations, or tobacco-control organisations were included in the study. In addition, a number of newspaper articles, which detailed tobacco-industry influencing strategies on SP, were identified through online searches and are cited in the text. These represented important secondary data sources in cases where journalists had access to information and documents relating to tobacco industry activities otherwise unavailable in the public domain.

Semi-structured interviews were also undertaken within the context of a wider study of tobacco-control developments in Europe and tobacco industry political strategies to influence policy processes. Interviews were conducted with government ministers and officials from national governments, officials from the European Commission, Members of the European Parliament, public health advocates and other civil society actors engaged in the policy process. BH undertook 17 interviews related to tobacco-control issues at the EU level in Brussels between September 2014 and December 2016 and 15 interviews in Dublin, Edinburgh and via Skype between October 2015 and October 2016 to examine policy developments at the national level and the role of the Irish government in the conclusion of the TPD during its Presidency of the Council of the EU in 2014. Skype interviews included representatives of the Australian tobacco-control community, but not actors engaged in Uruguayan policy. This reflects both the practical and linguistic challenges of undertaking such interviews and the principal focus of the book on SP.

Interviewees were identified through purposive sampling via a review of documents relating to the TPD and the plans to introduce SP in Ireland, and through online searches of actors and organisations engaged in these policy debates and processes. 'Snowballing' was employed to identify further potential informants from interviewees. Interviews were recorded, transcribed and coded by BH using NVivo 10 qualitative data analysis software. This involved an initial review of the transcripts to identify key themes and topics. These were noted during the first reading of transcripts and formed the basis of the codebook developed for the more systematic coding of transcripts in the second reading. Key themes were set up as 'nodes' and transcripts uploaded to NVivo for coding. During the analysis process, new codes emerged and previously identified codes were modified, combined and deleted as greater familiarity with the data continued to develop our understanding and interpretation of policy processes and the interconnections between different aspects of these. Following the coding, BH assembled a list of key findings. CH concurrently reviewed the audio recordings; the reliability of the coding, the analysis of the data and the publication strategy were then agreed in discussion between BH and CH. The latter included the analysis of the emergence of SP in Europe at the EU and member-state levels examined in the current volume, as well as a separate article examining the globally coordinated strategies of TTCs across a range of jurisdictions (Hawkins et al. 2018), which provides some of the context for the present volume. The first draft of the manuscript was produced by BH. CH then commented on and edited the draft, which was then revised by BH. SM drafted the literature review and discussion chapters, following discussion with BH and CH. The entire manuscript was then edited iteratively by CH and BH prior to publication. Interview data quoted here is not exhaustive, but key quotations are selected to represent wider points evident from the interview and documentary analysis.

The Structure of This Book

The outline of the book is as follows. The next chapter sets out the theoretical underpinning for the analysis we present. Chapter 3 examines the development of the EU TPD. We draw on both previously published material and new primary data collected in this study, principally from interviews conducted with policy actors in Ireland, the UK and Brussels, to examine the ways in which tobacco industry actors sought to prevent or delay the adoption of the Directive, and to remove proposals for SP and minimise compulsory labelling requirements in its final contents. Chapter 4 examines the overlapping yet distinct policy developments on SP in Ireland. In addition, it examines the horizontal interconnection between policy debates in Ireland and the UK and the vertical interconnection between developments at the national and EU levels. Chapter 5 shifts the focus from the tobacco industry to the public health community. It examines the role of international NGO networks, particularly the connections between tobacco-control advocates in Australia, Ireland and the UK in facilitating the introduction of SP laws, initially in Ireland and subsequently in the UK and other member states. Given the importance of public health actors' efforts to resist industry strategies to block and undermine SP, the policy learning which occurred between civil society actors in different settings is of vital importance in understanding policy dynamics in the area of tobacco packaging. Chapter 6 discusses the theoretical implications of our findings and the conclusions to be drawn from this work by scholars, public health actors and policy-makers.

The ordering of the chapters reflects both the chronology of events—in which the EU TPD was concluded before the introduction of SP at the member-state level—and the underlying logic of the policy process. The TPD played a key role in facilitating the introduction of SP at the national level; Article 22(4) of the TPD authorises national governments to adopt additional packaging restrictions in areas not covered by common action at the EU level. This provided an important political incentive and legal cover for governments considering such measures. Consequently, policy processes at the EU level (Chapter 3) are examined before those at the national level (Chapter 4). We also examine policy developments in Ireland and industry attempts to oppose these before examining transnational NGO networks and their role in policy transfer (Chapter 5). This reflects the analytical focus of Chapter 5 on the policy-making, legislative and implementation phases of the policy process rather than the agenda-setting phase. While the example of Australia was vital in bringing SP onto the policy agenda at the EU level, as well as in member states such as Ireland and the UK, our focus is not on the role of the Australian tobacco-control community as policy entrepreneurs, but as policy *facilitators* supporting the successful introduction of SP once it had been identified by European governments as a policy objective.

Bibliography

Bero, L. A. (2005). Tobacco industry manipulation of research. *Public Health Reports, 120*(2), 200–208.

Bertollini, R., Ribeiro, S., Mauer-Stender, K., & Galea, G. (2016). Tobacco control in Europe: A policy review. *European Respiratory Reviews, 25*, 151–157.

Brandt, A. M. (2012). Inventing conflicts of interest: A history of tobacco industry tactics. *American Journal of Public Health, 102*, 63–71.

CFTFKs. (2018). *The Global Cigarette Industry*. Centre for Tobacco-Free Kids. Available at https://www.tobaccofreekids.org/assets/global/pdfs/en/Global_Cigarette_Industry_pdf.pdf. Accessed 9 February 2019.

Chapman, S., & Freeman, B. (2014). *Removing the emperor's clothes: Australia and tobacco plain packaging*. Sydney: Sydney University Press.

Fooks, G., Smith, J., Lee, K., & Holden, C. (2017). Controlling corporate influence in health policy making? An assessment of the implementation of Article 5.3 of the World Health Organization Framework Convention on Tobacco Control. *Globalization and Health, 13*, 597.

Gilmore, A. B. (2012). Understanding the vector in order to plan effective tobacco control policies: An analysis of contemporary tobacco industry materials. *Tobacco Control, 21,* 119–126.

Gilmore, A. B., Branston, J. R., & Sweanor, D. (2010). The case for OFSMOKE: How tobacco price regulation is needed to promote the health of markets, government revenue and the public. *Tobacco Control, 19*(5), 423–430.

Gneiting, U., & Schmitz, H. P. (2016). Comparing global alcohol and tobacco control efforts: Network formation and evolution in international health governance. *Health Policy Plan, 31*(1), i98–i109.

Hafez, N., & Ling, P. M. (2005). How Philip Morris built Marlboro into a global brand for young adults: Implications for international tobacco control. *Tobacco Control, 14,* 262–271.

Hawkins, B., & Holden, C. (2016). A corporate veto on health policy? Global constitutionalism and investor-state dispute settlement. *Journal of Health Politics, Policy and Law, 13,* 1–19.

Hawkins, B., & Holden, C. (2018). European union implementation of article 5.3 of the framework convention on tobacco control. *Globalization and Health, 14,* 79.

Hawkins, B., Holden, C., Eckhardt, J., & Lee, K. (2016). Reassessing policy paradigms: A comparison of the global tobacco and alcohol industries. *Global Public Health.* https://doi.org/10.1080/17441692.2016.1161815.

Hawkins, B., Holden, C., & Mackinder, S. (2018). A multi-level, multi-jurisdictional strategy: Transnational tobacco companies' attempts to obstruct tobacco packaging restrictions. *Global Public Health.* https://doi.org/10.1080/17441692.2018.1446997.

Henriksen, L. (2012). Comprehensive tobacco marketing restrictions: Promotion, packaging, price and place. *Tobacco Control, 21,* 147–153.

Hervey, T. K. (2001). Community and national competence in health after tobacco advertising. *Common Market Law Review, 38*(6), 1421–1446.

Holden, C., & Hawkins, B. (2013). 'Whisky gloss': The alcohol industry, devolution and policy communities in Scotland. *Public Policy & Administration, 28*(3), 253–273.

Holden, C., & Lee, K. (2009). Corporate power and social policy: The political economy of the transnational tobacco companies. *Global Social Policy, 9*(3), 328–354.

Holden, C., & Hawkins, B. (2017). Law, market building and public health in the European Union. *Global Social Policy,* 1–17.

Hurt, R. D., Ebbert, J. O., Muggli, M. E., Lockhart, N. J., & Robertson, C. R. (2009). Open doorway to truth: Legacy of the Minnesota tobacco trial. *Mayo Clinic Proceedings, 84*(5), 446–456.

Jarman, H. (2015). *The politics of trade and tobacco control.* Basingstoke: Palgrave Macmillan.

McKee, M., Hervey, T., & Gilmore, A. (2010). Public health policies. In E. Mossialos, G. Permanand, R. Baeten, & T. Hervey (Eds.), *Health systems governance in Europe: The role of European Union law and policy* (pp. 231–281). Cambridge: Cambridge University Press.

Neuman, M., Bitton, A., & Glantz, S. (2002). Tobacco industry strategies for influencing European Community tobacco advertising legislation. *Lancet, 359*(9314), 1323–1330.

Olivet, C., & Villareal, A. (2016, July 28). Who really won the legal battle between Philip Morris and Uruguay? *The Guardian*. Available at https://www.theguardian.com/global-development/2016/jul/28/who-really-won-legal-battle-philip-morris-uruguay-cigarette-adverts. Accessed 1 March 2019.

Peeters, S., Costa, H., Stuckler, D., McKee, M., & Gilmore, A. B. (2015). The revision of the 2014 European Tobacco Products Directive: An analysis of the tobacco industry's attempts to 'break the health silo'. *Tobacco Control*. https://doi.org/10.1136/tobaccocontrol-2014-051919.

Savell, E., Gilmore, A. B., Fooks, G., & Derrick, G. E. (2014). How does the tobacco industry attempt to influence marketing regulations? A systematic review. *PLoS One, 9,* e87389. https://doi.org/10.1371/journal.pone.0087389.

Smith, K. E., Savell, E., & Gilmore, A. B. (2013). What is known about tobacco industry efforts to influence tobacco tax? A systematic review of empirical studies. *Tobacco Control, 22*(2), 144–153.

Voon, T., Mitchell, A., & Liberman, J. (Eds.). (2014). *Regulating tobacco, alcohol and unhealthy foods: The legal issues*. Abingdon: Routledge.

Weishaar, H., Collin, J., & Amos, A. (2016). Tobacco control and health advocacy in the European Union: Understanding effective coalition-building. *Nicotine & Tobacco Research, 18*(2), 122–129.

Wigand, J. (1996). *Jeffrey Wigand on 60 minutes*. Available at http://www.jeffreywigand.com/60minutes.php. Accessed 5 February 2019.

World Health Organization (WHO). (2003). *WHO framework convention on tobacco control* [Online]. Available at https://www.who.int/tobacco/framework/WHO_FCTC_english.pdf. Accessed 5 February 2019.

World Health Organization (WHO). (2008). *MPOWER: A policy package to reverse the tobacco epidemic*. Geneva: WHO.

World Health Organization (WHO). (2013). *Guidelines for implementation of the WHO FCTC*. Geneva, Switzerland: World Health Organization.

CHAPTER 2

Policy Transfer in the Context of Multi-level Governance

Abstract This chapter reviews the theoretical literature relating to the core concepts used in the study: multi-level governance and policy transfer. The evolution of the concept of policy transfer is traced through discussions of associated concepts such as policy diffusion, policy convergence, policy learning and lesson-drawing. It discusses the development of these ideas through the models of Dolowitz and Marsh, and Evans and Davies. Most importantly for this book, the chapter discusses developments in the literature that consider policy transfer beyond 'methodological nationalism'—the assumption that policy transfer involves bilateral lesson-drawing between states—to focus on the roles of international organisations and non-state actors.

Keywords Multi-level governance · Policy transfer · Policy learning · Corporations · Tobacco control

This chapter discusses the key concepts underpinning the analysis presented below and positions the book in relation to the relevant theoretical literature. We situate our study in relation to two main concepts from the political science and policy studies literature: multi-level governance and policy transfer. Policy transfer captures not only the movement and uptake

B. Hawkins et al., *The Battle for Standardised Cigarette Packaging in Europe*, Palgrave Studies in Public Health Policy Research,
https://doi.org/10.1007/978-3-030-31034-9_2

of policy *measures* across policy domains, but also the adoption of political strategies, arguments and ideas by policy actors in different settings via transnational policy networks. As will be argued below, policy transfer of standardised packaging (SP) to Europe was facilitated by precisely this type of policy learning, in particular among NGO actors in EU member states such as Ireland, whose successful campaigning for SP opened the way for the wider adoption of the policy elsewhere in the EU. First, though, we turn to the concept of multi-level governance, which explains the institutional context within the EU in which policy transfer and the contestation of policies takes place.

Multi-level Governance

The development of standardised tobacco packaging in Europe has to be seen within the specific policy-making context in which the policy developed. In Chapter 3, we discuss the specific institutional architecture of the EU and its decision-making processes as a prelude to our analysis of the passage of the 2014 Tobacco Products Directive (TPD). Here, it is sufficient to recognise that the EU represents a supranational level of political decision-making nested between national (and subnational) decision-making levels below it and global political structures above it (e.g. the United Nations [UN] and the World Trade Organization [WTO]).

The concept of multi-level governance (MLG) was developed in the context of European integration to understand and explain the processes of governing which emerge from decision-making at different levels, including—especially in the case of highly devolved member states such as Germany and Spain—the relevant sub-national authorities (Marks et al. 1996; Hooghe and Marks 2001; Marks and Hooghe 2004; Bache and Flinders 2004). Whilst studies of MLG seek to disaggregate between the different forms and loci of sub-national governance (e.g. cities and municipalities, local authorities, devolved administrations such as Scotland or powerful federal entities such as the German Länder; see for example Havlík and Kuchyňková 2017), our national-level case study is a small, centralised member state: Ireland. As such, we focus our analysis on the interactions between the national and supranational levels. Whilst we remain cognizant of the existence of sub-national decision-making, we do not attempt to differentiate between these entities and their treatment in the research literature. The governing treaties of the EU establish both certain areas of exclusive competence for the Union (e.g. the customs union and the common commercial policy; see Article 3 of the Treaty on the Functioning of the European Union [TFEU]) and shared competences (e.g. the internal market and related issues including social policy and public health; see Article 4 TFEU). Other areas are defined as national competences (e.g. culture, tourism and the protection and improvement of human health; see Article 6 TFEU), although the EU—whilst unable to pass legally binding measures—may act to support, coordinate or supplement national measures in these areas. In areas where the EU does not have exclusive competence, the interplay between EU and member-state competences is guided by the principle of subsidiarity (see Article 5(3) of the Treaty on European Union [TEU] and Protocol 2 TEU), which sets out the basis on which it should be decided whether policy decisions ought to be taken at the EU versus the national (or appropriate sub-national) levels. Paraphrasing somewhat, the principle of subsidiarity sets out that policy decisions ought to be taken at the lowest possible level, and thus as closely as possible to the citizens they will affect and govern. Only where common action at the EU level is needed to fulfil the obligations of the treaties should common action be taken at the EU level, thereby ensuring the regulatory autonomy of member states in relevant areas.

The complex system of MLG that has emerged (and continues to evolve) within the context of the European integration process has had significant consequences for policy-making and policy actors at all levels. Whilst it is obvious that the member states have shaped the evolution and development of the EU and the policies it pursues, the flow of influence is not unidirectional. EU membership has also shaped the internal politics of EU members. A now extensive literature on the 'Europeanization' of policy-making has examined the effects of EU membership on national (and sub-national) policies, polities and administrations within the member states (see Conzelmann 2008; Featherstone and Radaelli 2003; Bache and Jordan 2006; Börzel and Risse 2007; Radaelli 2008; Bache 2008; Warleigh-Lack 2008). Stephenson (2013) reviewed the contribution of the concept of MLG in the twenty years following its first mention in the research literature (see Marks 1993). He identified five distinct strands within the MLG literature, focusing on different aspects of MLG and linked to specific time frames in the development of this scholarship.

The first generation of studies arose (largely) in the context of the reformed EU structural and cohesion policies from 1988 and the '1992' project to complete the single internal market, focusing on the division of responsibilities between national and supranational entities in the administration of these complex policy mechanisms (see Marks et al. 1996; Scharpf 1997; Bache 1998; Hooghe and Marks 2001). In addition to the focus on the interaction between different levels of decision-making, this literature illuminated new *modes* of administration captured by the term governance (versus government), which implied a shift towards new forms of policy-making involving networks of experts, stakeholders and interest representation (Bache and Flinders 2004; Jessop 2004; Kohler-Koch and Eising 1999; Hooghe and Marks 2003). The second, 'functional', strand in the literature expanded analysis of MLG to new policy areas and policy-making settings largely via country case studies (Stephenson 2013). The third strand developed the focus on new modes of governance offering more radical interpretations of the decentred and network-based form of policy-making and implementation represented by the EU and the evolving forms of policy instruments to which these gave rise (see Hodson and Maher 2001; Kaiser and Prange 2004; Schmitter and Kim 2005). The fourth component of the literature identified by Stephenson focuses on the normative dimension of MLG, particularly the issues of legitimacy, democracy and accountability raised by the new modalities and territorialities of the national and supranational governance emerging within the EU (Olsson 2003; Peters and Pierre 2004; Harlow and Rawlings 2006; Hooghe and Marks 2008). Stephenson's final strand in the literature focuses on the current phase of scholarship on MLG which has sought to develop and apply the concept beyond the EU context in which it first evolved, examining the WTO and the UN systems (Knodt 2004; Enderlein 2010; Kaul 2010) and the functioning of public–private partnerships within these wider institutional contexts (Beisheim et al. 2010). Others meanwhile have applied the concept of MLG to forms of regional integration outside of Europe, e.g. in Asia, North America and the former Soviet Union (de Prado 2007; Sbragia 2010; Schreurs 2010; Obydenkova 2010).

The concept of MLG has also been applied in policy areas of direct relevance to the subject of the current volume. Chatwin (2007) used the concept to analyse drug policy within the EU and its member states, identifying widely varying policy approaches and health outcomes and identifying MLG not only as a valuable analytical concept, but as offering a potential model for future policy development. Lang and Rayner (2005) meanwhile examined the (then) emerging EU-level competence in nutrition and obesity policy and the implications for national-level governance, calling for coordinated European-level action to tackle the emerging crisis. Asare et al. (2009) analysed tobacco-control policy in the UK within the wider context of EU membership, focusing on the role of the subnational devolved administrations (i.e. the Scottish government) in policy development. They concluded that theories of MLG provide better explanations of policy development compared to alternative theories of regulatory federalism, highlighting the evolving authority for different aspects of tobacco-control policy within this:

> Over the past two decades the UK government's monopoly on all tobacco policy has been replaced by shared control among three levels of government. The central state now shares authority with the EU for policies on taxation, health warnings, advertising and tobacco contents. It has also devolved responsibility on health education, smoking cessation strategies, and indoor non-smoking regulation to Scotland, Wales and Northern Ireland. (Asare et al. 2009: 96)

Mamudu and Studlar (2009) have employed the concept of MLG to understand the negotiation and ratification process of the WHO Framework Convention on Tobacco Control (WHO 2003; see also Cairney et al. 2012; Studlar 2009).

Mavrot and Sager (2018) examine the issue of smoking cessation policy in Switzerland, a highly decentralised federal system, through the concept of vertical epistemic communities (see also Studlar et al. 2011 on 'vertical policy diffusion'). Smoking cessation advocates were able to influence policy at the federal level through coordinated influencing activities, building on policy developments at, and sharing of best practice from, the Cantonal level. They highlight the key role of both horizontal and vertical networks in influencing policy debates:

> The existing need for horizontal and vertical coordination in such systems provides these networks with numerous opportunities to promote their views. By including the key players at different levels (national and subnational civil servants for instance), experts in the vertical epistemic communities are able to diffuse their solution in many policy arenas and to play with the different levels, as Studlar (2009) has shown, in order to avoid deadlock. (Mavrot and Sager 2018: 404)

Whilst their case study is drawn from a small, national (albeit strongly federal) political community, the authors explicitly identify the relevance of their work for studies of different multi-level polities, including the US and the EU.

MLG is thus not only an established paradigm for understanding policy and regulatory dynamics within the EU and its member states, it has also been applied specifically to the issue of tobacco-control policy both in the EU and other multi-level (federal) polities (e.g. see Studlar 2008, on US tobacco control). The current volume builds on the existing literature by taking a MLG perspective in order to understand and explain attempts to introduce SP in Europe, initially at the EU level and subsequently within member states such as Ireland, in which prior developments at the EU level played a key facilitating role in the implementation of SP. However, our analysis is not Eurocentric and we place developments in that continent in the context of global tobacco-control policy debates and developments. In particular, we focus on the key role of policy advocates and transnational advocacy networks within this process. We recognise the indebtedness of tobacco-control advocates in Europe to their colleagues in Australia, the first country in the world to legislate for SP. Consequently, we combine our focus on vertical networks and knowledge exchange with a consideration of horizontal policy transfer and advocacy networks which operated between Australia and Ireland. To conceptualise these processes we need to engage with a further body of literature. To this end, the following sections of this chapter situate the current study in the context of previous studies of policy diffusion and transfer.

Policy Diffusion

The 1960s and 1970s saw the first studies of, and attempts to theorise, the spread and adoption of policies across the federal system in the US and then internationally (Walker 1969; Gray 1973). Berry and Berry (1999: 171) defined diffusion as 'the process by which an innovation is communicated through certain channels over time among members of a social system'. Dobbin et al. (2007) outline four distinct theories, which seek to explain the causal mechanisms by which diffusion occurs: the *constructivist* school, the *coercion* school, the *economic competition* school and the *learning* school.

The constructivist school argues that an increasingly global 'political culture' generates a broad consensus over the efficacy of policies, and that the ideas underpinning policies are socially constructed. Therefore, it is changes in *ideas* within this global political culture that generate changes in policies; countries are affected by global norms (Boli-Bennett and Meyer

1978). Understanding policy change thus requires us to understand how the ideas underpinning certain policies become socially accepted. Dobbin et al. (2007) highlight three ways in which policy change may occur: (a) the leading countries act as 'exemplars' for other countries to follow; (b) 'specialists' make arguments about a policy's appropriateness or applicability to another policy setting (often based on perceived similarities between countries) (Strang and Meyer 1993); or (c) expert groups 'theorise' the effects of a policy, providing a rationale for its adoption. 'Expert theorisation' has formed the basis of a significant body of work on the role of international organisations in policy diffusion processes; expert theorisation has been categorised by DiMaggio and Powell (1983) as 'normative isomorphism', and scholars such as Finnemore and Sikkink (2001) have demonstrated how international organisations and governments have used this mechanism by constructing theories of action and efficacy.

The *coercion* school is based on the idea of changes in incentives. It identifies how countries may be driven to adopt particular policy approaches by external stimuli. For example, conditionality mechanisms put in place by international organisations can *coerce* countries into adopting a particular policy. 'Softer' mechanisms of 'coercion' include the impact of hegemonic ideas or powerful policy leadership on policy decisions, demonstrating that, even without direct power structures and material incentives, dominant global actors are able to influence policy discourses and implementation through 'ideational' channels (Gruber 2000). Therefore, certain actors hold a disproportionate amount of power.

The *economic competition* school argues that policy diffusion is brought about by the need to remain economically competitive in the global market place. For a state to flourish, it must match its competitors in choosing market-friendly policies. Finally, the *learning* school identifies the belief systems of policy-makers as the key factor driving policy change. This school argues that diffusion does not occur through reaction to external environments, but rather when policy-makers' beliefs are changed through the production of new evidence (Dobbin et al. 2007). Like the constructivist school, the learning school attributes policy diffusion to the power of ideas. Again, international organisations can play a part here, as their powerful research capability and their networks for dissemination of evidence mean they are able to channel learning.

Different disciplines, including sociology, political science and economics, have developed different theories of policy diffusion that often speak to an identical 'phenomenon' (Dobbin et al. 2007). However, a common theme across disciplines is that policy often spreads through 'percolation' or 'contagion' rather than as the result of a conscious choice (Stone 2004), and is often dispersed through the dissemination of an idea or practice from an external source. Various diffusion streams have been empirically identified through the literature, including national communication networks through state officials, geographical proximity between jurisdictions, connections between 'leader' versus 'laggard' states and vertical influence through national government systems (Berry and Berry 1999).

Theories of diffusion were criticised for failing to explain how policies were adapted or changed during the diffusion process (Orenstein 2003; Stone 2004, 2012). In addition, it was argued that they relegated agency within the theory, prioritising instead the conditions necessary for diffusion and the mechanisms by which policies spread. Policy diffusion was therefore presented as a process of osmosis, rather than as an action-oriented intentional process with decision-making dynamics (Evans 2009; Dolowitz and Marsh 1996). In response to this, a plethora of agency-centred approaches appeared, with a vast array of nomenclature that created conceptual confusion around the processes of diffusion and policy change (Stone 2004). These included 'lesson-drawing' (Rose 1991, 1993), 'bandwagoning' (Ikenberry 1990), 'policy learning' (May 1992) and 'social learning' (Hall 1993). Dolowitz and Marsh (1996, 2000) used the umbrella term of 'policy transfer' to encompass the different conceptualisations that were emerging.

Policy Transfer

Dolowitz and Marsh (1996) were amongst the first scholars to develop a comprehensive agency-centred theory of policy transfer. They argued that policy transfer occurs as 'a result of strategic decisions taken by actors inside and outside of government' (1996: 343). They believed that the different conceptualisations of diffusion theory, policy learning and lesson-drawing identified above were not in fact competing theories, but rather 'different dimensions' of the policy transfer process (Hudson and Lowe 2009). Drawing particularly on the work of Rose on 'lesson-drawing' (1991, 1993) and Bennett on 'policy convergence' (1991), they created the most widely cited definition of policy transfer as:

> … a process in which knowledge about policies, administrative arrangements, institutions etc. in one time and/or place is used in the development of policies, administrative arrangements and institutions in another time and/or place. (Dolowitz and Marsh 1996: 344)

They highlighted two important dimensions of transfer: *voluntary transfer*, which occurs through direct choice and agency of transfer actors, and *coercive transfer*, where a government or supranational agency forces another government to adopt a particular policy that is in their interests, explicitly highlighting the importance of agency (or lack thereof) in their framework. This created a 'middle ground' between the diffusion theorists, with their lack of attention to agency, and newer conceptualisations, which saw policy transfer only as a voluntary act performed by rational actors.

Dolowitz and Marsh's framework developed a 'map' of the process of transfer through a series of questions, which focused 'on the relationship between voluntary and coercive (forced) transfer and the links between policy transfer and policy "success" or failure' (2000: 6). The series of questions that provided the heuristic framework for this map were as follows:

1. *Why do actors engage in policy transfer?* Putting the distinction between voluntary and coercive transfer at the centre of this question, Dolowitz and Marsh (1996, 2000) argue that voluntary transfer is the result of some form of dissatisfaction or problem with the status quo. Perceived policy 'failure' creates incentives to identify new policies that can be borrowed from elsewhere. Coercive transfer, while rarer, comes about through supranational mechanisms such as international treaties, trade and investment agreements, or the actions of international organisations such as the World Bank or International Monetary Fund (IMF). As will be explored in more detail below, the European Union is an important actor in this regard. Transnational corporations are also able to exert coercive pressure for policy change, through their ability to threaten to 'take their business elsewhere' (see Farnsworth [2004] for an extended treatment of this point). Indirect coercive transfer can be forced upon governments through externalities, such as environmental damage, or through technological progress or economic integration, which compel governments to work together to solve supranational problems.

2. *Who are the key actors involved in the policy transfer process?* Dolowitz and Marsh (1996, 2000) identify nine categories of transfer actors, some directly involved in the transfer process, and some who are external 'influencers': elected officials; political parties; bureaucrats/civil servants; pressure groups; policy entrepreneurs and experts; transnational corporations; think tanks; and supranational governmental and non-governmental institutions and consultants. This final group has gained a particular power in recent years—this will be returned to later, as scholars such as Stone (2004, 2012) have done much to show how decision-making powers have been moving away from national elected bodies in recent years.
3. *What is transferred?* Dolowitz and Marsh (1996, 2000) seek to move away from narrow conceptualisations of policy transfer, which focus only on policy goals and instruments (see Bennett 1991) and instead seek to incorporate broader macro objects of transfer such as ideology, ideas, and negative lessons.
4. *From where are lessons drawn?* The origins of policy lessons are key to the 'multi-level' nature of enquiry that encapsulates Dolowitz and Marsh's (1996) model. They argue that policy actors can turn to different levels of governance—the international, national and local—to draw inspiration, which provides opportunities for both horizontal transfer (between nations, geographical areas or sectors) and vertical transfer (through different levels of governance). Evans and Davies (1999) build on this model, as discussed below.
5. *What are the different degrees of transfer?* Dolowitz and Marsh (2000) offer a spectrum of policy transfer, from 'copying' at one end of the scale to 'inspiration' at the other, where policy-makers do not adopt all aspects of a policy or seek to achieve identical outcomes.
6. *What restricts or facilitates the policy transfer process?* Following Rose (1991), Dolowitz and Marsh (1996, 2000) emphasise that policies are not imported into a vacuum, and the contextual, institutional and political arrangements of the borrowing jurisdiction and the specific motivations and objectives of decision-makers influence the success or failure of policy implementation.
7. *How is the process of policy transfer related to policy "success" or policy "failure"?* Closely related to Question 6, Dolowitz and Marsh (2000) identify three elements of the transfer process that are critical for 'successful' transfer outcomes: information deficit, 'cherry-picking' and contextual factors. If a borrowing jurisdiction does not have full

information about the policy itself and the institutional arrangement within which it sits, this leads to 'uninformed' transfers. Where a policy, and the institutional aspects that make it a success, are not transferred in their entirety, then there is the risk of 'incomplete' transfer. Finally, the differences between the original and borrowing jurisdiction can result in 'inappropriate' transfer.

Dolowitz and Marsh's (1996, 2000) model was praised for creating a comprehensive framework that incorporated many different types of transfer, and which addressed those processes more holistically, encompassing both coercive and voluntary mechanisms of transfer while acknowledging both the causes and impacts of policy outcomes (Benson and Jordan 2011; Evans 2009, 2010). However, it also faced criticism of its status as a mere heuristic device rather than an explanatory theory of policy change (James and Lodge 2003; Evans and Davies 1999). Evans and Davies (1999) sought to address these weaknesses by incorporating five different approaches to policy change—international structure and agency; domestic structure and agency; policy network analysis; policy transfer analysis; and epistemic community approaches—into a single theoretical model addressing both structural and agency-related aspects of policy transfer. In addition, they focus on the 'spatial' dimension of policy transfer within and between different levels of governance. They identify 25 transfer pathways, working *horizontally* and *vertically* between the five different levels of governance (the transnational, regional, international, national, and local levels). They argue that economic, technological, ideological and institutional structures of the 'borrowing' and 'lending' jurisdictions must be analysed in order to establish how they facilitate policy transfer, and the impact on the transfer process. The focus on the supranational dimension also draws attention to the ways in which international and transnational forces impact the institutions and processes of policy transfer.

The model draws on the policy network (Marsh and Rhodes 1992a, b) and epistemic communities (Adler and Haas 1992) literature to analyse the process through which decision-makers 'acquire and utilize knowledge' (Evans and Davies 1999: 376). The resulting model consists of several stages, which break down the transfer process into discrete actions:

- *Recognition*: whereby a decision-making elite, politician or bureaucrat (known as the 'client') identifies a policy problem;

- *Search*: which is undertaken if an obvious acceptable policy response is not available;
- *Contact*: whereby a policy transfer 'agent' (for example an epistemic community within an international organisation) is identified;
- *Emergence of an information feeder network*: whereby the 'client' is provided with an increase in volume and detail of information regarding the potential for transfer;
- *Cognition, reception and the emergence of a transfer network*: whereby the client evaluates the information provided by the information feeder network, with cognition and reception depending on a common value system existing between the client and the network;
- *Elite and cognitive mobilisation*: whereby the transfer agent's information and networks are tested, as they are expected to provide robust information on programmes or policies that address similar problems to those experienced by the client at the 'recognition' stage;
- *Interaction*: whereby the transfer agent organises forums for the exchange of ideas between the client and knowledge elites with policy-relevant knowledge;
- *Evaluation*: whereby the client evaluates the intelligence gathered by the agent relating to the object of transfer (e.g. policy goals, content, instruments, institutions, ideology), the degree of transfer (e.g. copying, hybridisation or inspiration) and the prerequisites of transfer (e.g. political feasibility and institutional conditions);
- *Decision*: whereby the chosen policy is tested against other competing ideas arising in the borrowing jurisdiction, within what Kingdon (1984) describes as the 'policy primeval soup';
- *Implementation*: whereby the policy is adopted by the client country, often by implementers who are different people to those who formulated the policy.

International and Global Perspectives on Policy Transfer

Since Dolowitz and Marsh (1996) established policy transfer as an analytical focus, the concept has been developed to create a wide and varied body of literature that has been combined with a range of other theories and concepts to categorise and explain processes of transfer within and between political jurisdictions and contexts. Benson and Jordan (2011) identify three major approaches within this literature. One has sought to promote policy transfer as a means of stimulating policy innovation (Rose 2005). The second has looked to develop theories around policy transfer, and the third has applied these theoretical developments to new empirical avenues, such as social and welfare policy (Pierson 2003), crime (Jones and Newburn 2006), and development assistance (Stone 2004). This has turned the study of policy transfer and change into a multidisciplinary field that has moved far beyond its origins in comparative public policy. International relations scholars, for example, have developed theories on policy diffusion, whereas political economy scholars have concentrated on structural factors concerning the institutional architecture of jurisdictions that generate convergence. The engagement with the wider conceptual literature has seen policy transfer linked to policy networks (Stone 2004, 2012), to theories of epistemic communities (Hulme 2005; Dunlop 2009), and presented as an incremental, chaotic process whereby ideas are 'nicked from all over the place' (Dwyer and Ellison 2009).

While most studies acknowledge the influence of external international forces, Stone (2004, 2012) argues that the majority of policy transfer studies suffer from a 'methodological nationalism' that excludes a thorough interrogation of these international forces and their influence within the national (or sub-national) policy-making spheres:

> The very words 'policy transfer' implies a direct exchange process between exporting and importing countries with an implicit tendency to assume a bilateral relationship. (Stone 2012: 490)

Evans (2004) identifies the emergence of new opportunity structures for influencing agents, by highlighting the 'hollowing out' of the state both externally (through globalisation) and internally (through the privatisation and marketisation of public services), and the shift from traditional to collaborative governance. Globalising forces, therefore, such as the growth of international markets and the transnationalisation of corporate structures, have not only altered the channels through which domestic policy actors can seek policy ideas, but also broadened the 'pool' of actors involved in the policy process to include networks and organisations at the international and global levels.

Stone (2004, 2012) has led the effort to integrate international and transnational forces into theoretical frameworks for policy transfer and associated concepts, drawing attention to mechanisms embedded in markets and policy networks and examining the role of international and transnational actors in these processes. She draws attention to 'soft' forms of transfer, such as the spread of norms and knowledge, as an important complement to the traditional focus of 'hard' transfer of policies, institutions and programmes which are the key focus of the mainstream policy transfer literature. The potential for transnational policy transfer, however, does not necessarily result in convergence between countries, as negative lessons can be learned that result in divergence: 'the policy transfer literature therefore allows us to see possibilities for convergence around policy objectives and principles but divergence with regard to instruments adopted, types of legislation, or institutional modes of control and delivery' (Stone 2012: 485). In placing transnational forces at the heart of policy transfer analysis, therefore, Stone (2004, 2012) emphasises the conceptual importance of policy *learning*, which in turn requires the acknowledgement and potential redefinition of the interests that can affect the fundamental ideas or attitudes to policy mechanisms.

Stone's (2004, 2012) work has sought to correct the 'methodological nationalism' in the traditional transfer literature by broadening the understanding of *where* transfer takes places and *who* is involved in it. She seeks to redress the horizontal intergovernmental focus of much of the literature to incorporate ideas around multi-level governance, and in so doing create a model that acknowledges vertical policy transfer between national and supranational policy venues. She argues for a more dynamic, transnational perspective on policy transfer, which analyses the interactions between states, international organisations and non-state actors.

Transnational Non-state Actors

Stone (2004, 2012) argues that the field of policy transfer suffers from its own terminology and, more specifically, the emphasis this places on 'policy' as opposed to the transfer of the ideas, behaviours and perceptions that form the normative context within which policies are transferred. If the transfer framework is broadened to consider these concepts, then actors such as NGOs or social movements become critical transfer actors. Drawing on the literature on transnational advocacy frameworks (Keck and Sikkink 1999), she argues that NGOs and social movements can become actors within the policy environment, playing key advocacy and agenda-setting roles within particular policy arenas (Stone 2004). Additionally, policy transfer can be achieved by mechanisms embedded within global market structures beyond the national sphere.

Stone (2004) identifies a key role for 'policy entrepreneurs' as transnational transfer actors, which facilitate the exchange between different actors and act as 'resource' banks through which policy discourses and ideas can spread through professional networks. The first of these policy entrepreneur groups are transnational think tanks, which act as independent policy analytical bodies outside of state structures, and have become a model of transfer through their empirical lesson-drawing approach (Stone 2004, 2012). A second policy entrepreneur group is philanthropic foundations, such as the Bill & Melinda Gates Foundation, which have spread norms and procedures from American culture throughout the world. The final group is multinational consultants, who, for example, were influential in institutionalising New Public Management (NPM) around the world by creating a 'fashion-setting' expert network at a time when governments were turning to external consulting services.

The involvement of non-state actors in policy-making and transfer processes has led to what Stone (2004, 2012) calls the 'transnationalisation' of policy, whereby the policy process is no longer the sole prerogative of national governments or international organisations. Rather, the proliferation of actors has resulted in the incorporation of social and—importantly—corporate interests into the 'primeval soup' of the policy-making environment (Kingdon 1984). The capacities and motivations of the different non-state actors vary, which complicates the analysis of transfer, particularly if the analysis is broadened to include the ideational aspects of 'soft' transfer. Stone (2004) points out that how ideas structure thinking and how they become institutionalised are important, but complex, aspects of policy analysis; this is a particularly important consideration in an analysis of how transnational tobacco corporations interact with policy transfer processes, as this broadening of the focus of transfer and the consideration of transnational actors opens up many more entry points within the transfer process where both TTCs and public health NGOs are potentially able to interact with other important actors and to influence the discourse.

Furthermore, analysis that pays attention to how states, international organisations and non-state actors interact, and puts the locus of attention onto the collaborative pursuit of policy solutions, draws attention to new modes of governance that shift the policy debate away from the traditional forums of state actors, epistemic communities or advocacy networks. These formations of policy collaboration also provide opportunities for transnational corporations to shape the debate. Stone (2004, 2012) highlights three such collaborative mechanisms: the first is 'soft law and private regulatory standards' (Stone 2012), which have become an important mechanism of voluntary or non-state regulation, but which in some contexts have been taken up enthusiastically by transnational corporations as a way of avoiding legally binding state regulations and shaping the discourse of regulation in their favour, as has been demonstrated for the alcohol industry (Holden and Hawkins 2016). The second form of policy collaboration is 'global policy partnerships' (Stone 2012), such as the Paris Convention on Climate Change, which are often initiated by international organisations such as the UN to address global problems but are implemented at the national level.

The final form of policy collaboration are what Stone (2004) calls 'global public policy networks' (GPPNs) such as the 'Roll Back Malaria Initiative', whereby a multiplicity of actors engage within a network to address a particular policy area. Stone (2004) points out that GPPNs are distinct from epistemic communities as the latter situate themselves as groups of scientific authority, and thereby exclude activist groups, which can be an important feature of GPPNs. Similarly, GPPNs are distinct from transnational advocacy groups, which are concerned with agenda setting and advocacy, whereas GPPNs have more 'delegated' authority from states and international organisations. This authority grants them the status of a governance structure (unlike epistemic communities and transnational advocacy networks). As a network, GPPNs facilitate 'soft' transfer by representing 'an informal and gradual mode for the international dissemination of ideas and policy paradigms ... participants can build alliances, share discourses and construct the consensual knowledge that defines an international policy community' (Stone 2004: 560). They can also facilitate 'hard' transfer of policies due to their mode of transnational governance, and can generate regulation, coordination, the pooling of authority and decision-making processes.

The linkages between the participants in a GPPN form a governance structure outside the hierarchical modes of national or international organisational governance. Networks, Stone (2004) argues, therefore act as both agents and structures, and incorporating them into transfer analyses helps to reconcile the agent-centred bias of the transfer literature with the analysis of structural considerations seen in the diffusion and convergence bodies of scholarship. Furthermore, these 'formal' networks and the associated governance structures provide further opportunities for transnational corporations to enter the debate and shape it in a way that maximises their interests. However, as we noted in the introductory chapter of this book, and in contrast to many other transnational corporations, TTCs have been excluded from a number of policy networks, although they continue to use broader organisations such as cross-industry associations to press their interests. They may therefore find it more difficult than other transnational corporations to exploit some formal GPPNs, at least when openly acting on their own behalf. Nevertheless, multi-level governance structures have opened up new avenues of influence for well-organised corporations such as TTCs, and we return to the analysis of such multi-level structures in the next sub-section.

International Organisations and Multi-level Governance

Much of the literature on international organisations such as the World Bank and the IMF focuses on their coercive power, such as the IMF's use of conditionality to push governments to bring their economic policies into line with the 'Washington Consensus' (e.g. Vreeland 2003; Mosley et al. 1995). Similarly, they have considerable power over the production and dissemination of ideas, which can shape policy.

The EU is unique among international organisations in terms of its law-making and enforcement powers. The policy transfer literature highlights how the EU's model of multi-level governance offers multiple, highly developed and effective channels for policy transfer, including:

- 'Borrowing' policy ideas from member states (Héritier 1996);
- The negotiation of common rules;
- Acting on treaty powers, for example through CJEU jurisprudence (Bulmer et al. 2007);
- Implementing treaty obligations;
- Through the Open Method of Coordination (Bomberg and Peterson 2000).

Radaelli (2000) was one of the first to apply policy transfer theory to the EU, conceptualising it as a 'massive transfer platform'. Drawing on sociological institutionalism, advocacy coalition frameworks and analysis of epistemic communities, he argues that policy ideas emerge from the more dominant countries within the EU (such as Germany and the UK) and become embedded through EU institutions, particularly the Commission. He identifies three isomorphic processes through which common polices become embedded in national political systems via EU institutions:

- *Coercive isomorphic processes*, where the EU uses its authority to force nation states to converge around policy programmes;
- *Mimetic isomorphic processes*, where uncertainty and the need for legitimacy drive countries to copy policies in place in other states perceived to be more successful or legitimate;
- *Normative isomorphic processes*, where epistemic communities exchange information and policy ideas through the EU's structures and activities on the basis of shared experiences, identities and cognitive schemata.

Bomberg and Peterson (2000) take an 'agency-centred' approach to the EU, presenting it as a 'supranational idea hopper' and focusing on the voluntary mechanisms within the EU, in particular the horizontal governance mechanism of the Open Method of Coordination (OMC), which is designed to encourage the exchange of ideas between nation states. Looking at policy tools such as agreements, peer reviews and the identification of best practice, they argue that the voluntary mechanisms of transfer have the potential to enhance the EU's legitimacy, and build consensus and trust, through the forum the EU provides to encourage the translation of policies through the different levels of European governance.

Bulmer and Padgett (2005) use an institutional approach in their analysis, focusing on the structural elements to examine the context in which rational actors search for policies. They argue that the EU as a polity presents three different institutional contexts, which generate different transfer processes and outcomes. The first institutional context is governance by negotiation, namely the process by which EU policy is adopted through the Council of Ministers of the EU. Polices are agreed by common consent, and consequently there are opportunities for member states to 'upload' their policy preferences to a supranational level. The majority vote system results in a largely voluntary process of transfer, although those countries that do not vote with the majority will face coercion. The second institutional context is governance by hierarchy, where powers are promoted to the supranational level, and ideas are subsequently 'downloaded' to the national level. This coercive approach is supported by judicial mechanisms, whereby laws are available to enforce obligation. The final institutional context is governance by facilitation, where national policy-makers interact within EU settings. Sovereignty consequently remains with the domestic polities, but transfer occurs 'horizontally' between the different nations, representing an entirely voluntary, unilateral process of transfer.

Most studies of policy transfer within the EU focus on transfer between the different institutional levels of the union and between member states. We note, however, that studies of interest representation within the EU have identified that large firms take advantage of multi-level systems by operating simultaneously at different levels and utilising a range of channels to access policy-makers, and generally have greater resources to do so than citizens' groups (Coen 1997, 2007; Bouwen 2002; Dur and Mateo 2012). Such studies focus on lobbying and the use of litigation by corporations, and have not been considered in the context of policy transfer. In this book, we explicitly consider the role of corporations, examining how their strategies impact upon the transfer activities of policy-makers and public health advocates, and how the various actors adapt, respond and attempt to counter each other in their efforts to facilitate or block policies. One aspect of this process, of particular importance to the analysis of systems of multi-level governance, is the potential ability of interest groups to venue shift (Mazey and Richardson 2006; Coen 2007), that is, to move decision-making on an issue from one setting or level to another where they are more likely to achieve their desired outcome. Baumgartner and Jones (1991) argue that successful venue-shifting involves a process of redefinition of the 'policy image', a process others have referred to as 're-framing' (Hawkins and Holden 2013). We note that these policy 'images', or 'frames', can also be transferred from one setting to another, alongside substantive policies. The choice of frames is thus an important part of any struggle over the content of a policy, the venue(s) within which it is shaped, and whether it is ultimately adopted or not.

Policy Transfer and Tobacco Control

There is a small sub-set of literature that looks specifically at tobacco control and policy transfer. Studlar (2006) highlights five policy instruments within the field of tobacco control—regulation, economic incentives, public education, capacity building (e.g. funding for community development programmes) and general learning tools (e.g. the release of tobacco industry documents). Drawing on theories of convergence, globalisation and policy emulation he identifies three 'families' of states within advanced industrial economies that have experienced similar policy trajectories and outcomes in tobacco control. The first is the 'Anglo-American' family of Canada, the US, Australia and New Zealand, who have demonstrated since the 1980s similar policy pathways on issues such as health warnings on packets and standardised packaging, taxation, restrictions on advertising and marketing, underage sales and environmental smoke regulations. Studlar (2006) highlights various examples of emulation, such as the elimination or reduction of subsidies to tobacco producers, or controls over environmental tobacco smoke. Three of these countries, Canada, Australia and the US, pioneered the first International Treaty for Smoke-Free Flights in 1994, a policy quickly adopted throughout the aviation industry.

Delving deeper into the transfer and convergence relationships between these countries, Studlar (2006) identifies certain institutions, particularly federalism (all but New Zealand have federalist governments), that have advantages in terms of gaining traction for tobacco control within the political agenda, due to the increased availability of policy-making jurisdictions which results in greater potential for 'venue-shopping' by public health advocates. The type of federalism is important—the US has lagged behind Canada and Australia in tobacco control due to more veto points within the American system, which allow tobacco interests to block central legislation. In addition to federalist mechanisms, Studlar (2006) also identifies developing cultures (as opposed to traditional culture) around 'secular morality', whereby emerging ideas around public health and desirable public behaviour become a 'key ingredient' in explaining the rapid policy transfer and converging mechanisms for tobacco control among these leaders of policy in this field.

The second 'family' of countries that Studlar (2006) identifies is the Scandinavian countries (excepting Denmark, which sits in the third family), which were early leaders in the use of policy instruments such as advertising bans, educational campaigns, strong warning labels and taxation. Studlar (2006) points to their close cultural outlook, the similar presentation of problems associated with tobacco and their established institutions of cooperation such as the Nordic Council as the mechanisms by which they present similar models of tobacco control. The third 'family' consists predominantly of the original members of the EU; the UK, France, Germany, Italy, Ireland and Denmark, which chose instruments such as the banning of TV advertising and sponsorship, mandated warning labels, minimum taxation levels and tar maximums. These policies came through EU directives, which member states then transposed into legislation.

Cairney (2007) draws on advocacy coalition framework and punctuated equilibrium theories, complemented with ideas from multi-level governance and policy transfer scholars, to create an explanation of policy change within the UK. He calls for close attention to historical narratives of policy, arguing that they are crucial to explanatory models of policy change. As an example he highlights the 'dominance narrative' around tobacco-control policy development in the UK, which emphasises post-war stability and inertia, and argues that the recent changes to tobacco policies were only made possible by changes to existing network relationships through globalisation and the development of the EU. This dominance narrative posits that the discourse in the post-war period was driven by the definition of tobacco as an economic issue, whereby public health concerns were all but excluded from the policy networks and policy was formed around self-regulation approaches until external influences were exerted. In contrast, the 'incremental narrative' of tobacco-control policy change argues that the policies followed established trajectories, and external forces had little effect on policy change; science and health concerns were not excluded to the extent suggested by the 'dominance narrative', and regulation was inevitable if the self-regulation route of tobacco control failed. Cairney (2007), therefore, argues for a 'multiple lenses' approach, whereby different models are applied to a case study rather than vice versa, in order to give a more complete explanation of policy change.

Summary

Reviewing the development of the policy transfer literature, Benson and Jordan (2011) highlight how the traditional focus on 'hard' transfer mechanisms such as goals, targets and instruments has broadened to include 'soft' elements of transfer, including the exchange of ideas, ideologies and belief systems. The locus of transfer scholarship, they argue, has moved away from its government-centric emphasis focused on horizontal transfer between national policy contexts to include multi-level and multi-actor accounts of policy transfer. This provides an apt description of the literature that neatly summarises the key importance of MLG structures, non-state actors and a broad approach to what may be transferred. In the next three chapters, we present our empirical findings on the battle for strengthened cigarette packaging requirements in Europe, focused at the EU level, at the national level, and on the role of civil society actors, respectively. In the final chapter, we analyse these findings in light of the concepts discussed in this chapter.

Bibliography

Adler, E., & Haas, P. (1992). Conclusion: Epistemic communities, world order, and the creation of a reflective research program. In P. Haas (ed.), *Knowledge, power and international policy coordination*. A Special Issue of *International Organisation, 46*(1), 367–390.

Asare, B., Cairney, P., & Studlar, D. T. (2009). Federalism and multilevel governance in tobacco policy: The European Union, the United Kingdom, and devolved UK institutions. *Journal of Public Policy, 29*(1), 79–102.

Bache, I. (1998). *Politics of European Union regional policy: Multi-level governance or flexible gatekeeping?* Sheffield: Continuum.

Bache, I. (2008). *Europeanization and multilevel governance: Cohesion policy in the European Union and Britain*. Lanham, MD: Rowman & Littlefield.

Bache, I., & Flinders, M. (2004). Multi-level governance and the study of the British state. *Public Policy and Administration, 19*(1), 31–51.

Bache, I., & Jordan, A. (Eds.). (2006). *The Europeanization of British politics*. London: Palgrave Macmillan.

Baumgartner, F., & Jones, B. (1991). Agenda dynamics and policy subsystems. *The Journal of Politics, 53*(4), 1044–1074.

Beisheim, M., Campe, S., & Schäferhoff, M. (2010). Global governance through public-private partnerships. In H. Enderlein, S. Wälti, & M. Zürn (Eds.), *Handbook on multi-level governance* (pp. 370–382). Cheltenham: Edward Elgar.

Bennett, C. J. (1991). What is policy convergence and what causes it? *British Journal of Political Science, 21*(2), 215–233.

Benson, D., & Jordan, A. (2011). What have we learned from policy transfer research? Dolowitz and Marsh revisited. *Political Studies Review, 9*(3), 366–378.

Berry, F. S., & Berry, W. D. (1999). Innovation and diffusion models in policy research. In P. A. Sabatier (Ed.), *Theories of the policy process* (pp. 169–200). Boulder, CO: Westview Press.

Boli-Bennett, J., & Meyer, J. (1978). The ideology of childhood and the state: Rules distinguishing children in national constitutions, 1870–1970. *American Sociological Review, 43*, 797–812.

Bomberg, E., & Peterson, J. (2000). *Policy transfer and Europeanization: Passing the Heineken Test?* (Queen's Papers on Europeanisation p0002). Queen's University Belfast.

Börzel, T., & Risse, T. (2007). Europeanization: The domestic impact of European Union politics. In K. E. Jorgensen, M. A. Pollack, & B. Rosamond (Eds.), *Handbook of European Union politics* (pp. 483–504). Thousand Oaks: Sage.

Bouwen, P. (2002). Corporate lobbying in the European Union: The logic of access. *Journal of European Public Policy, 9*(3), 365–390.

Bulmer, S., Dolowitz, D., Humphreys, P., & Padgett, S. (2007). *Policy transfer in European Union governance: Regulating the utilities.* London: Routledge.

Bulmer, S., & Padgett, S. (2005). Policy transfer in the European Union: An institutionalist perspective. *British Journal of Political Science, 35*(1), 103–126.

Cairney, P. (2007). A "multiple lenses" approach to policy change: The case of tobacco policy in the UK. *British Politics, 2*(1), 45–68.

Cairney, P., Studlar, D., & Mamudu, H. (2012). *Global tobacco control: Power, policy, governance and transfer.* London: Palgrave Macmillan.

Chatwin, C. (2007). Multi-level governance: The way forward for European illicit drug policy? *International Journal of Drug Policy, 18*(6), 494–502.

Coen, D. (1997). The evolution of the large firm as a political actor in the European Union. *Journal of European Public Policy, 4*(1), 91–108.

Coen, D. (2007). Empirical and theoretical studies in EU lobbying. *Journal of European Public Policy, 14*(3), 333–345.

Conzelmann, T. (2008). A new mode of governing? Multi-level governance between cooperation and conflict. In T. Conzelmann & R. Smith (Eds.), *Multi-level governance in the European Union: Tasking stock and looking ahead* (pp. 11–30). Baden-Baden: Nomos.

de Prado, C. (2007). *Global multi-level governance: European and East Asian leadership.* Tokyo: United Nations University Press.

DiMaggio, P. J., & Powell, W. W. (1983). The iron cage revisited: institutional isomorphism and collective rationality in organizational fields. *American Sociological Review, 48,* 147–160.

Dobbin, F., Simmons, B., & Garrett, G. (2007). The global diffusion of public policies: Social construction, coercion, competition, or learning? *Annual Review of Sociology, 33,* 449–472.

Dolowitz, D., & Marsh, D. (1996). Who learns what from whom: A review of the policy transfer literature. *Political Studies, 44*(2), 343–357.

Dolowitz, D., & Marsh, D. (2000). Learning from Abroad: The role of policy transfer in contemporary policy-making. *Governance, 13*(1), 5–23.

Dunlop, C. A. (2009). Policy transfer as learning: Capturing variation in what decision-makers learn from epistemic communities. *Policy Studies, 30*(3), 289–311.

Dur, A., & Mateo, G. (2012). Who lobbies the European Union? National interest groups in a multilevel polity. *Journal of European Public Policy, 19*(7), 969–987.

Dwyer, P., & Ellison, N. (2009). 'We nicked stuff from all over the place': Policy transfer or muddling through? *Policy & Politics, 37*(3), 389–407.

Enderlein, H. (2010). Economic policy-making and multi-level governance. In H. Enderlein, S. Wälti, & M. Zürn (Eds.), *Handbook on multi-level governance* (pp. 423–440). Cheltenham: Edward Elgar.

Evans, M. (Ed.). (2004). *Policy transfer in global perspective*. Abingdon: Routledge.

Evans, M. (2009). Policy transfer in critical perspective. *Policy Studies, 30*(3), 243–268.

Evans, M. (Ed.). (2010). *New directions in the study of policy transfer*. Abingdon: Routledge.

Evans, M., & Davies, J. (1999). Understanding policy transfer: A multi-level, multi-disciplinary perspective. *Public Administration, 77*(2), 361–385.

Farnsworth, K. (2004). *Corporate power and social policy in a global economy*. Bristol: Policy Press.

Featherstone, K., & Radaelli, C. (Eds.). (2003). *The politics of Europeanization*. Oxford: Oxford University Press.

Finnemore, M., & Sikkink, K. (2001). Taking stock: The constructivist research program in international relations and comparative politics. *Annual Review of Political Science, 4,* 391–416.

Gray, V. (1973). Innovation in the states: A diffusion study. *American Political Science Review, 67,* 1174–1185.

Gruber, L. (2000). *Ruling the world: Power politics and the rise of supranational institutions*. Princeton, NJ: Princeton University Press.

Hall, P. (1993). Policy paradigms, social learning and the state: The case of economic policy making in Britain. *Comparative Politics, 25,* 275–297.

Harlow, C., & Rawlings, R. (2006). *Promoting accountability in multi-level governance: A network approach* (European Governance Papers).

Havlík, V., & Kuchyňková, P. (2017). Cities and regions in competition? Negotiations for the 2014–2020 programming period in the Czech Republic. *Transylvanian Review of Administrative Sciences, 13*(50), 90–109.

Hawkins, B., & Holden, C. (2013). Framing the alcohol policy debate: Industry actors and the regulation of the UK beverage alcohol market. *Critical Policy Studies, 7*(1), 53–71.

Héritier, A. (1996). The accommodation of diversity in European policy-making and its outcomes: Regulatory policy as a patchwork. *Journal of European Public Policy, 3,* 149–167.

Hodson, D., & Maher, I. (2001). The open method as a new mode of governance: The case of soft economic policy coordination. *Journal of Common Market Studies, 39*(4), 719–746.

Holden, C., & Hawkins, B. (2016). Health policy, corporate influence and multi-level governance: The case of alcohol policy in the European Union. In N. Kenworthy, R. Mackenzie, & K. Lee (Eds.), *Case studies on corporations and global health governance: Impacts, influence and accountability* (pp. 145–158). London: Rowman & Littlefield.

Hooghe, L., & Marks, G. (2001). *Multi-level governance and European integration.* Oxford: Rowman & Littlefield.

Hooghe, L., & Marks, G. (2003). Unraveling the central state, but how? Types of multi-level governance. *American Political Science Review, 97*(2), 233–243.

Hooghe, L., & Marks, G. (2008). A postfunctionalist theory of European integration: From permissive consensus to constraining dissensus. *British Journal of Political Science, 39,* 1–23.

Hudson, J., & Lowe, S. (2009). *Understanding the policy process: Analysing welfare policy and practice* (2nd ed.). Bristol: Policy Press.

Hulme, R. (2005). Policy transfer and the internationalisation of social policy. *Social Policy & Society, 4*(4), 417–425.

Ikenberry, G. J. (1990). The international spread of privatization policies: Inducements, learning and "policy band wagoning". In E. Suleiman & J. Waterbury (Eds.), *The political economy of public sector reform and privatization.* Boulder, CO: Westview Press.

James, O., & Lodge, M. (2003). The limitations of 'policy transfer' and 'lesson drawing' for public policy research. *Political Studies Review, 1*(2), 179–193.

Jessop, B. (2004). Multi-level governance and multi-level metagovernance. In I. Bache & M. Flinders (Eds.), *Multi-level governance* (pp. 49–74). Oxford: Oxford University Press.

Jones, T., & Newburn, T. (2006). *Policy transfer and criminal justice.* Milton Keynes: Open University Press.

Kaiser, R., & Prange, H. (2004). Managing diversity in a system of multi-level governance: The open method of co-ordination in innovation policy. *Journal of European Public Policy, 11*(2), 249–266.

Kaul, I. (2010). The changing role of the United Nations: Lessons for multi-level governance. In H. Enderlein, S. Wälti, & M. Zürn (Eds.), *Handbook on multi-level governance* (pp. 323–342). Cheltenham: Edward Elgar.

Keck, M. E., & Sikkink, K. (1999). Transnational advocacy networks in international and regional politics. *International Social Science Journal, 51*(159), 89–101.

Kingdon, J. W. (1984). *Agendas, alternatives and public policies.* Boston, MA: Little, Brown.

Knodt, M. (2004). International embeddedness of European multi-level governance. *Journal of European Public Policy, 11*(4), 701–719.

Kohler-Koch, B., & Eising, R. (Eds.). (1999). *The transformation of governance in the European Union.* London: Routledge.

Lang, T., & Rayner, G. (2005). Obesity: A growing issue for European policy? *Journal of European Social Policy, 15*(4), 301–327.

Mamudu, H. M., & Studlar, D. T. (2009). Multilevel governance and shared sovereignty: European Union, member states, and the FCTC. *Governance, 22*(1), 73–97.

Marks, G. (1993). Structural policy and multi-level governance in the EC. In A. Cafruny & G. Rosenthal (Eds.), *The state of the European Community: The Maastricht debate and beyond* (pp. 391–411). Lynne Reinner: Boulder, CO.

Marks, G., & Hooghe, L. (2004). Contrasting visions of multi-level governance. In I. Bache & M. Flinders (Eds.), *Multi-level governance* (pp. 15–30). Oxford: Oxford University Press.

Marks, G., Hooghe, L., & Blank, K. (1996). European integration from the 1980s: State-centric v Multi-level governance. *Journal of Common Market Studies, 34*(3), 341–378.

Marsh, D., & Rhodes, R. A. W. (1992a). New directions in the study of policy networks. *European Journal of Political Research, 21,* 181–205.

Marsh, D., & Rhodes, R. A. W. (1992b). *Policy networks in British government.* Oxford: Clarendon Press.

Mavrot, C., & Sager, F. (2018). Vertical epistemic communities in multilevel governance. *Policy & Politics, 46*(3), 391–407.

May, P. J. (1992). Policy learning and failure. *Journal of Public Policy, 12*(4), 331–354.

Mazey, S., & Richardson, J. (2006). Interest groups and EU policy-making: Organisational logic and venue shopping. In J. Richardson (Ed.), *European Union: Power and policy-making.* Abingdon: Routledge.

Moseley, P., Harrigan, J., & Tove, F. J. F. (1995). *Aid and power: The World Bank and policy-based lending* (Vol. 1). London: Routledge.

Obydenkova, A. (2010). Multi-level governance in post-Soviet Eurasia: Problems and promises. In H. Enderlein, S. Wälti, & M. Zürn (Eds.), *Handbook on multi-level governance* (pp. 292–307). Cheltenham: Edward Elgar.

Olsson, J. (2003). Democracy paradoxes in multi-level governance: Theorizing on structural fund system research. *Journal of European Public Policy, 19*(2), 283–300.

Orenstein, M. (2003). Mapping the diffusion of pension innovation. In R. Holzmann, M. Orenstein, & M. Rutkowski (Eds.), *Pension reform in Europe: Process and progress.* Washington, DC: World Bank.

Peters, B., & Pierre, J. (2004). Multi-level governance and democracy: A Faustian bargain? In I. Bache & M. Flinders (Eds.), *Multi-level governance* (pp. 75–89). Oxford: Oxford University Press.

Pierson, C. (2003). Learning from labor? Welfare policy transfer between Australia and Britain. *Commonwealth and Comparative Politics, 41*(1), 169–186.

Radaelli, C. (2000). Policy transfer in the European Union: Institutional isomorphism as a source of legitimacy. *Governance, 13*(1), 25–43.

Radaelli, C. (2008). Europeanization, policy learning, and new modes of governance. *Journal of Comparative Policy Analysis, 10*(3), 239–254.

Rose, R. (1991). What is Lesson-Drawing? *Journal of Public Policy, 11*(1), 3–30.

Rose, R. (1993). *Lesson drawing in public policy: A guide to learning across time and space*. Chatham, NJ: Chatham House.

Rose, R. (2005). *Learning from comparative public policy: A practical guide*. London: Routledge.

Sbragia, A. (2010). Multi-level governance and comparative regionalism. In H. Enderlein, S. Wälti, & M. Zürn (Eds.), *Handbook on multi-level governance* (pp. 267–278). Cheltenham: Edward Elgar.

Scharpf, F. (1997). Introduction: The problem-solving capacity of multi-level governance. *Journal of European Public Policy, 4*(4), 520–538.

Schmitter, P., & Kim, S. (2005). The experience of European integration and the potential for Northeast Asian integration. *East-West Center Working Papers, 10*, 1–23. Available at https://www.eastwestcenter.org/sites/default/files/private/PSwp010.pdf. Accessed 9 February 2019.

Schreurs, M. (2010). Multi-level governance the ASEAN way. In H. Enderlein, S. Wälti, & M. Zürn (Eds.), *Handbook on multi-level governance* (pp. 308–320). Cheltenham: Edward Elgar.

Stephenson, P. (2013). Twenty years of multi-level governance: 'Where does it come from? What is it? Where is it going?' *Journal of European Public Policy, 20*(6), 817–837.

Stone, D. (2004). Transfer agents and global networks in the 'transnationalization' of policy. *Journal of European Public Policy, 11*(3), 545–566.

Stone, D. (2012). Transfer and translation of policy. *Policy Studies, 33*(6), 483–499.

Strang, D., & Meyer, J. W. (1993). Institutional conditions for diffusion. *Theory and Society, 22*, 487–511.

Studlar, D. T. (2006). Tobacco control policy instruments in a shrinking world: How much policy learning? *International Journal of Public Administration, 24*(4–6), 367–396.

Studlar, D. T. (2008). US tobacco control: Public health, political economy, or morality policy? *Review of Policy Research, 25*(5), 393–410.

Studlar, D. T. (2009). Tobacco control policy in Western Europe: A case of protracted paradigm change. In G. Capano & M. Howlett (Eds.), *European and North American policy change: Drivers and dynamics* (pp. 91–110). Abingdon: Routledge.

Studlar, D. T., Christensen, K. & Sitasari, A. (2011). Tobacco control in the EU-15: The role of member states and the European Union. *Journal of European Public Policy, 18*(5), 728–745.

Vreeland, J. R. (2003). *The IMF and economic development*. New York: Cambridge University Press.

Walker, J. (1969). The diffusion of innovation among the American states. *American Political Science Review, 63*, 880–899.

Warleigh-Lack, A. (2008). The EU, ASEAN and APEC in comparative perspective. In P. Murray (Ed.), *Europe and Asia: Regions in Flux* (pp. 23–41). Basingstoke: Palgrave Macmillan.

World Health Organization (WHO). (2003). *WHO framework convention on tobacco control* [Online]. Available at https://www.who.int/tobacco/framework/WHO_FCTC_english.pdf. Accessed 5 February 2019.

CHAPTER 3

The EU Tobacco Products Directive

Abstract This chapter presents the study's findings in relation to the development, negotiation and adoption of the European Union's 2014 Tobacco Products Directive, focusing on the activities of transnational tobacco companies (TTCs) in attempting to block, amend and/or delay the passage of the Directive within the European Union's institutions. It analyses the political strategies of TTCs, and those of third parties acting for them, in lobbying the European Commission, the European Parliament and member states within the Council of the European Union.

Keywords EU Tobacco Products Directive · European Commission · European Parliament · Council of the European Union · Transnational tobacco companies

The European Union's (EU's) 2014 Tobacco Products Directive (TPD) attempted to respond to scientific and political developments in the field of tobacco control since the adoption of the previous directive (2001/37/EC) in 2001. Above all, the Directive sought to meet the EU's obligations as a signatory of the World Health Organization's (WHO's) Framework Convention on Tobacco Control (FCTC). In addition, it responded to technological developments in the industry by putting forward a regulatory regime for electronic cigarettes (e-cigarettes). Following

B. Hawkins et al., *The Battle for Standardised Cigarette Packaging in Europe*, Palgrave Studies in Public Health Policy Research,
https://doi.org/10.1007/978-3-030-31034-9_3

an internal process, the European Commission published a formal proposal for the Directive in December 2012. In June 2013 the Council of the European Union ('the Council') adopted its position on the Commission proposal, while the European Parliament (EP) also considered it under the EU's Ordinary Legislative Procedure. Following the committee stage, the EP adopted its position and gave a negotiating mandate to lead Member of the European Parliament (MEP) Linda McAvan to enter 'trialogue' negotiations with the Commission and the Council. Political agreement on the text of the Directive was announced in December 2013 before the Directive was formally adopted by the EP and Council in February and March 2014, respectively. It entered into force in May 2014, with a deadline of May 2016 for member states to transpose it into national law.

The provisions of the TPD presented a comprehensive challenge to the business model of the global tobacco industry which, as indicated in Chapter 1, is highly dependent on branding and promotion, and market segmentation through product differentiation and carefully targeted pricing structures. Acknowledging the key role these factors play in recruiting and retaining smokers, the TPD sought to target the ability of TTCs to use the remaining channels available to them for consumer marketing. In particular, the Directive sought to target products, and characteristics of these, designed to recruit new smokers (see Table 3.1). These measures related principally to the packaging requirements for cigarettes and flavourings. Proposals included a minimum pack size of 20 cigarettes—and equivalent restrictions on minimum sale quantities for loose (or 'roll your own') tobacco leaf—to increase the price of the smallest quantities of cigarettes available and thus reduce entry points into smoking. In addition, small rectangular cigarette packs—often dubbed 'lipstick style' packaging—which target young women, a key demographic for the tobacco industry, were prohibited and standard packaging sizes introduced. Flavourings, including menthol, were to be banned on the grounds that they mask the taste and the throat irritation experienced by new smokers and thus smooth the transition into smoking. During the legislative process, e-cigarettes emerged as a new tobacco-control issue and measures were proposed for a dual-track approach in which they could be regulated either as medical devices or as tobacco products under the TPD. Of most relevance to the present discussion were the proposals on labelling and packaging requirements. Previous studies indicate that the Commission, during the preparatory stages of the legislative process, considered including standardised packaging (SP) in the proposed Directive, but this

Table 3.1 Key provisions of the EU Tobacco Products Directive (2014/40/EU)

Article	*Provision*	*Details*
Article 3	Maximum emission levels for tar, nicotine, carbon monoxide (10 mg) and other substances	Tar: 10 mg/cigarette Nicotine: 1 mg/cigarette Carbon monoxide: 10 mg/cigarette
Article 5	Reporting of ingredients and emissions	Manufacturers and importers must provide competent authorities in member states with – A list of all ingredients and quantities used in the manufacture of the tobacco products – The emission levels of substances referred to in Article 3 and, where available, information on other emissions and their levels
Article 7	Regulation of ingredients	Member states shall prohibit the placing on the market of tobacco products with a characterising flavour
Article 9	General warnings and information messages on tobacco products for smoking	Each packet of any tobacco product must carry one of two specified general warnings and an information message set out in the Directive in a standardised format and typeface
Article 10	Combined health warnings for tobacco products for smoking	Each packet must carry one of the text warnings listed in the Directive Annex I and a corresponding colour photograph specified in the picture library in Annex II in a set format and typeface These must cover over 65% of both the external front and back surface of the unit packet and any outside packaging

(continued)

Table 3.1 (continued)

Article	*Provision*	*Details*
Article 13	Product presentation	Product information that may suggest a product is less harmful to consumers or the environment, or refers to the smell or flavour of products, is banned Products that resemble foods or cosmetics are banned Labelling information on nicotine, tar and carbon monoxide is banned
Article 14	Appearance and content of unit packets	Packets may be cardboard or soft but must be cuboid in shape and contain at least 20 cigarettes (or 3 mg of rolling tobacco)
Article 15	Traceability	Member states must ensure that all unit packets of tobacco products are marked with a unique identifier
Article 18	Cross-border distance sales of tobacco products	Member states may (but are not obliged to) prohibit cross-border distance sales of tobacco products to consumers. Member states shall cooperate to prevent such sales
Article 20	Electronic cigarettes	Member states must follow a detailed regulatory framework for e-cigarettes whereby they can either regulate them as tobacco products under conditions set out in the Directive, or as medical devices
Article 24	Free movement (standardised packaging)	The Directive does not affect the right of member states to maintain or introduce further requirements for the standardisation of the packaging of tobacco products, where it is justified on grounds of public health

was omitted from the draft text eventually put forward to the EP and the Council (Peeters et al. 2015). Instead, the Directive significantly increased the size of mandatory health warnings (including graphic images) to cover 65% of the pack. Whilst the TPD stopped short of introducing mandatory SP requirements across the single market, it included an explicit acknowledgement that member states had the right to go beyond the minimum requirements set out in the Directive and to introduce SP unilaterally at the national level. This was a crucial development for national policy debates, providing a strong rationale for national governments to act unilaterally, or perhaps, more accurately, removing a potential reason for them not to proceed and a potential argument for industry actors to use to oppose policy development within member states.

There was a clear consensus amongst interview respondents from different sectors that packaging requirements, and warning labels, were of central importance for the TTCs. The industry strategy on the Directive has been widely discussed by public health actors and has received significant media attention, in part due to the leaking into the public domain of internal company documents that set out the lobbying strategy of one firm, Philip Morris International, and documents released under freedom of information (FOI) laws and analysed by researchers (Peeters et al. 2015). Estimations of the human and financial resources dedicated by the tobacco industry to the TPD vary, but all speak to a remarkable level of engagement in terms of the number of personnel dedicated to this and the budgets available to them. Philip Morris International (PMI) alone is thought to have spent €1.65m and employed over 160 lobbyists to work on the Directive (Peeters et al. 2015). This was the largest, and most extensive, lobbying campaign ever mounted against a piece of European legislation (European Ombudsman 2016). The lengths to which the TTCs were prepared to go to prevent the TPD demonstrate the degree of concern they had about its potential effects on their business model. Somewhat ironically from the industry perspective, the vehemence of the industry response to the TPD underlined the degree to which the TPD was feared by the industry, suggesting additional evidence for the effectiveness of the proposed measures in reducing cigarette consumption.

The industry strategy on the TPD can be easily summarised. As was revealed in the leaked PMI strategy documents (Hörz 2014; Peeters et al. 2015), their aim was to amend the provisions of the Directive and delay its adoption for as long as possible, whilst seeking to block the most far-reaching or 'extreme' proposals, identified as standardised packaging, a ban on certain ingredients and an end to point-of-sale displays of cigarettes (Peeters et al. 2015). This 'block, amend, delay' strategy was in keeping with the well-documented history of tobacco industry strategy to oppose potentially damaging regulations. As one interview respondent working in the public health sector commented, 'I don't think that the aims of the industry have changed in the meantime. So basically, they try to kill the TPD, delay or weaken it'. What was noteworthy in this instance was the granular level of detail with which the industry pursued its strategy, mapping for example the positions of each individual MEP on tobacco-control issues and their likely openness to overtures from the industry.

The ability to delay legislation was particularly important in the context of the political timetables of the EU institutions at the time in which the Directive was being prepared and debated. With EP elections scheduled for May 2014 and a new Commission to be appointed thereafter, the ability to delay the legislation through any means at this juncture could have meant the legislation would fall or would have to be reintroduced in the next Parliament. The potentially different political make-up in the EP, and different personnel in the Commission, may have meant that the proposal would not return or may have come back in a modified form less antithetical to industry interests. Delaying tactics were also important in the context of the rotating six-month presidency of the Council. The crucial stages of the legislative process on TPD were conducted under the Irish Council presidency in the first semester of 2013. Ireland, as will be discussed below, has a strong record as a leader on tobacco-control issues in Europe and had committed not just to the successful conclusion of the TPD, but to the introduction of SP domestically. Irish Health Minister James Reilly, who would chair the Health Council in this period, also demonstrated significant personal investment in the issue and a strong determination to see the Directive through. Tobacco-control advocates interviewed for this study agreed unanimously that the Irish Presidency, and Minister Riley in particular, were vital in securing the agreement on the Directive and feared that succeeding presidencies, which saw tobacco control as a lower priority, may have been unable to push it over the line.

The other key aspect of the industry strategy was the decision to work through third-party actors during the campaign, seeking to engage bodies from other sectors, which may have common interests with, or be amenable to the arguments of, the tobacco companies. As will be highlighted below,

TTCs engaged a wide range of outside actors and used different channels as the conduits for their positions in different contexts. Both aspects of their strategy demonstrate the capacity of the industry to take a highly nuanced approach, tailored to the political and institutional settings in which they are acting, and even tailoring their messaging and approach to the interests of specific individuals they are targeting.

The institutions of the EU remain at times hard to understand and navigate, even for those with a high degree of familiarity with them, although the tobacco industry's strategy in identifying key actors and junctures in the decision-making process demonstrates a highly sophisticated understanding of the policy context on their part. It is beyond the scope of this book to describe and explain in full detail the nuances of the EU legislative process. For the purposes of the analysis developed here it suffices to note that, since the entry into force of the Lisbon Treaty in 2009, the majority of EU legislation is now adopted according to the Ordinary Legislative Procedure set out in Article 294 of the Treaty on the Functioning of the European Union (TFEU). This involves a process of co-decision between the Commission, the European Parliament (EP) and the Council of the European Union, comprised of relevant ministers from member states, adopting decisions, in most instances, through qualified majority voting (QMV). The Commission retains the sole right of initiative, so all EU legislative processes begin with a proposal from the Commission, which is then sent to the EP and the Council for approval. In cases where there is agreement on all fronts, legislation may be adopted after the first reading. In cases where significant amendments are tabled by the EP or Council, or disagreements emerge between the institutions, a 'trialogue' process is convened between the three institutions which seeks to arrive at a compromise on the content of the bill before a second reading in the EP and the Council. At this stage, the legislation is either adopted (before or after a conciliation committee is needed to resolve tensions) or falls. TTCs sought to block, amend and delay the TPD across all three institutions and at all stages of the legislative process. The remainder of the chapter examines industry efforts to stymie the TPD. It is structured around the key institutions and actors involved in the EU legislative process and the specific industry strategies at each stage of the process. Each section includes a discussion of the specific role of each body in EU policy-making, in order to understand the specific strategies employed by the tobacco industry in each instance.

The Commission

It is a core tenet of political strategy that the most effective way to prevent or shape legislation is to intervene in the process at the earliest possible stage. The ability to set agendas, to dictate what issues come onto the table for discussion, and in what form, has long been recognised by political scientists as a key component of the exercise of political power (Bachrach and Baratz 1962; Lukes 1974). For corporate political actors seeking to shape policy agendas and the content of proposals, the Commission is, therefore, a key strategic target. The Commission is perhaps one of the least well understood yet most widely discussed bodies in the EU's complex institutional architecture. It is the target of much speculation and the source of many myths about the aims of the Union. Emanating from the French rather than the Anglo-Saxon administrative tradition, it is a hybrid entity combining aspects of both a civil service and an executive. It is more than a simple bureaucracy and less than an EU government, but executes certain functions of both. As indicated above, it is solely responsible for the generation of new legislative proposals, affording it great influence over the content of EU law. It is responsible also for the day-to-day running of the EU and, as 'guardian of the treaties', for the implementation and enforcement of the EU *acquis communautaire*.

Of relevance for the current discussion is the internal structure of the Commission and its organisation into different Directorates General (DGs), staffed by functionaries and focusing on specific areas of policy in ways analogous to government ministries and departments. Above the Commission services sits the College of Commissioners; political appointments made jointly by the member states and the EP and, in the person of the President especially, the public face of the Commission. The process through which legislative proposals emerge is complex and largely outwith the remit of the current book, but some appreciation of the internal structures and processes is necessary to fully appreciate the tobacco industry's influencing strategy on TPD. Proposals emerge in a specific DG, for example DG SANCO (now DG Santé; responsible for health and consumer affairs), and pass up through the different levels of that DG for revisions and amendment before being opened up to other components of the Commission for comment and potential revision, in a process known as the inter-services consultation. Proposals are also subject to other forms of oversight, including stakeholder consultation and regulatory impact assessment, before ultimately passing on to the College of Commissioners for final approval and publication.

The influence of industry actors over Commission deliberations has been documented elsewhere (Peeters et al. 2015; Costa et al. 2014; Berteletti et al. 2017). Interviewees for this study supported the conclusions of previous studies that the industry enjoyed significant access to the Commission during the crucial developmental stage of the Directive. As one representative of a non-governmental organisation (NGO), which monitored the development of the TPD closely, commented: 'what became very clear is that the tobacco industry had very easy access to the European Commission on the highest level'. Previous studies have detailed the extent of TTC access to the Commission at the very highest levels of the EU civil service and argued that the interventions of the former Commission Secretary General, Catherine Day, and Legal Service's Director-General, Luis Romero Requena, led to both significant delays in the progress of the TPD through the Commission structures and the removal of key proposals such as SP from the proposed Directive (Peeters et al. 2015). In keeping with previously identified industry tactics (Smith et al. 2010), the regulatory impact assessment was also used to delay the progress of the Directive. The Commission's public consultation, meanwhile, generated the highest number of responses ever recorded for a Commission proposal with over 85,000, many of which were the result of coordinated efforts by TTCs and third-party actors associated with them to overwhelm the Commission and stymie the progress of the proposed Directive (Tobacco Tactics 2016a).

The other key component to the industry strategy was to try to use the internal structure of the Commission, and the competing foci of different DGs, in an attempt to hollow out and delay the Directive. Whilst the objectives of the TPD were seen by DG SANCO as principally, if not uniquely, health-related, industry actors sought to engage other DGs whose portfolios were in some way relevant to, or affected by, the TPD, including DGs Enterprise, Trade, Agriculture and Rural Development and Internal Market (Peeters et al. 2015). These DGs, it could be assumed, would see the TPD in terms not simply of health but other issues such as jobs or tax revenue, which would be more in keeping with the industry's opposition to the proposals. In a move which would be mirrored in their approach to the key committees in the EP, the industry's divide-and-rule tactic between

DGs was designed to undermine the influence of the DG that was least sympathetic to them, and to dilute the proposals which they were politically able to put forward.

The industry's influencing strategy on the Commission was brought directly into the public consciousness with the emergence of the scandal involving Health Commissioner John Dalli. The scandal centred on alleged contacts between the Commissioner and Swedish Match, a producer of oral snuff ('snus') with links to Philip Morris, and the claims that associates of Dalli had solicited a bribe from the company on his behalf (Tobacco Tactics 2016b). The details of the case remain opaque and are widely contested, but some interview respondents, and wider commentaries on the incident and the TPD process, believed that the scandal was manufactured by the industry in a deliberate attempt to destabilise the Commission and thereby halt the progress of the Directive. The 'Dalligate' scandal has been recounted extensively elsewhere and the analysis presented here does not provide evidence of industry involvement beyond that which is already present in the public domain. Regardless of their role in the Dalli scandal, however, there is clear evidence that the industry was pursuing a more general strategy of delay. As one respondent stated:

> If there was [going to be] a Directive, it had to be adopted before the elections of 2014. And it was only possible if it would have been adopted during the Irish Presidency. So they did everything to delay [...]. It didn't work in the end in their advantage. But there was clearly a strategy. If it [sic] was no text being discussed in the Irish presidency, they did not have a Directive because that means it could not have been adopted before the elections. And then go to the next term with a new Commission, new Presidency. They would not have a Directive later on.

If the industry's intention was to delay, and thus derail, the Directive, it appears to have been a significant miscalculation on their part. The political controversy surrounding the case made engagement with the industry even more politically controversial than before. Following 'Dalligate', industry actors found non-health DGs less open to their overtures (Peeters et al. 2015). Moreover, rather than delaying the Directive as the industry may have hoped, the removal of Dalli created renewed impetus to conclude negotiations on the text. The official procedures to replace Dalli as Health Commissioner with his countryman Tonio Borg offered health advocates and MEPs committed to the TPD a chance to press home the case for its swift passage. In his confirmation hearings in front of the EP in November 2012, Borg's political commitment to TPD was made a prerequisite of his confirmation by MEPs. Borg was regarded by interviewees as a highly competent political operator and was commended for delivering on his promise of steering the TPD to adoption before the end of the 2009–2014 EP session. Borg's appointment facilitated a rapid process of adoption of the TPD, driven forward by the Irish Presidency of the Council.

The Member States and the Council

PMI leaked strategy documents reveal that national-level lobbying was a key component of the TTCs' strategy, and they used established links in member states in an attempt both to apply pressure to delay the proposed Directive by the Commission, via national delegations in Brussels, and to build a potential blocking majority in the Council to oppose key proposals and secure amendments (Peeters et al. 2015). Perhaps the hardest part of the EU legislative process to analyse are the deliberations between member states in the Council. In part at least, this is because Council meetings are held behind closed doors and are not minuted. In addition, the lobbying which occurs is also highly decentralised and occurs largely in national capitals to influence specific national governments' positions. As such, there is no central repository of information about engagement with the industry in terms of declarations of interests or logs of meetings with industry actors which, notwithstanding the limitations of these sources, exist in the public domain or are accessible via FOI requests for the Commission and the EP. To fully understand the dynamics of the Council negotiations and the positions it adopts would thus require significant efforts focusing at least on the main countries interested in the legislation and, ideally, on all relevant national policy debates. An exhaustive analysis of industry lobbying around member states is beyond the scope of this book. Instead we restrict ourselves to analysis of the key national actors and developments within the Council during the TPD's development.

In the case of the TPD, only four states—Romania, Bulgaria, the Czech Republic and Poland—opposed the adoption of the final Directive. This represented a significant break with past tobacco-control measures, which had been subject to far greater opposition from within the Council, including from some of the largest and most powerful member states. The decision of countries such as Germany—which has amongst the weakest tobacco-control laws in the EU, a politically influential domestic tobacco industry, and has opposed past measures to introduce tobacco-control policy at the EU level—to support the Directive reflects the current reluctance of national governments to oppose tobacco-control measures or to be seen to be pursing the interests of the tobacco industry over those of public health. Despite this, there were several additional countries which equivocated on the issue. Interview respondents indicated that countries expressing reservations about the TPD were those with domestic economic interests that may have been negatively affected by the TPD. These included not just those member states with cigarette production facilities, but others with domestic industries involved in the production of ancillary materials such as cigarette packaging.

The wider economic impacts of the TPD for associated industries reliant on tobacco consumption created potential opportunities for TTCs to engage national governments on their positions in the Council. Governments of countries with significant economic interests associated with the tobacco industry may be amenable to pursuing a tobacco industry agenda in multilateral forums such as the Council, as they seek to protect jobs and tax revenue. Moreover, engaging companies associated with, but independent from, tobacco producers avoided the controversy that surrounds the political influence of the tobacco industry and sidestepped issues associated with Article 5.3 of the FCTC. There is substantial evidence that TTCs have repeatedly used arguments about employment and tax revenues with governments to undermine support for tobacco-control policies, including on the issue of tobacco packaging (MacKenzie et al. 2018). Working through third parties was identified by PMI in its internal strategy documents as a key strategy for opposing the TPD, and is in keeping with the literature on TTC use of third-party actors in other settings (Tobacco Tactics 2016c, d). For companies in the TTCs' supply chain, there are clear incentives to promote the interests of their clients and oppose regulations that may affect tobacco sales and therefore their own businesses as well as those of the TTCS.

The European Parliament

The EP was perhaps the key institution in the TTCs' influencing strategy on the TPD. Leaked internal documents from PMI demonstrate a degree of detailed engagement with the EP commensurate with the significant financial and human resources deployed by the industry to oppose the Directive.

Individual MEPs were categorised using a colour-coding system to indicate their sympathy with TTC-amenable arguments and to engagement by the tobacco industry. Whilst influencing activities were directed across the member states and EU-level institutions, the significant legislative power granted to the EP under the Ordinary Legislative Procedure offered industry actors a key opportunity to delay and amend the Directive or to remove their least-favoured measures. In particular, the complex political landscape within the EP, in which the 736 MEPs balance party allegiance, national and regional concerns and the institutional interests of the EP itself (e.g. versus other institutions), creates an opportunity for policy actors to play off different groupings against one another and to target key structures and individuals in an attempt to shape agreements. As with most parliaments around the world, the EP works not only through plenary sessions of all members but through various committees and working groups, which debate and agree amendments before proposals are put to the plenary for institutional agreement. The passage of each piece of legislation through the EP is managed by a 'rapporteur'—an MEP from the lead committee on the portfolio—who is shadowed by designated MEPs from the other party groupings in the committee. Rapporteurs will also represent the EP in inter-institutional negotiations between the EP, the Council and the Commission. In the case of TPD, the lead committee was the Committee on Environment, Public Health and Food Safety (ENVI) and the rapporteur was British Labour Party MEP Linda McAvan, of the Progressive Alliance of Socialists and Democrats (S&D), who was shadowed by German MEP Karl-Heinz Florenz from the centre-right European People's Party (EPP).

With the passage of the TPD, the industry again demonstrated a detailed understanding of the workings of the Parliament and the potential for specific groups of actors to stymie the progress of the TPD at crucial junctures in the legislative process. Interviewees familiar with the parliamentary negotiations and the engagement of the industry in the EP indicate that representatives of TTCs enjoyed a high level of access to MEPs, despite the warnings about tobacco industry influence contained within the FCTC. As one respondent from the NGO sector commented:

> It became clear that the tobacco industry had very easy access to members of the European Parliament and that only a minority of the MEPs showed any form of caution in their contacts with the tobacco industry. And so, for both of those two institutions, the kind of approach that was – is recommended by – in the Tobacco Framework Convention and in Article 5.3.

This point was echoed by other respondents who highlighted the difficulty for MEPs in determining whether actors approaching them may be representing tobacco industry interests. As one interviewee working in the EU institutions commented:

> If you go up to the Parliament, there's a large amount of MEPs who were very happy to talk to the tobacco industry and then there's another large amount of MEPs who don't even know, and you know, again their lack of awareness but they would talk to associate groups.

A key aspect of the industry strategy in engaging MEPs was their ability to propose amendments to the legislation at the committee stage, which would have the potential effect of either weakening the proposals or, at the very least, delaying its progress through the EP. Lobbyists contacting MEPs with proposed amendments is a common and established feature of Brussels lobbying. In the case of the TPD, the involvement of the tobacco industry in co-ordinating proposed amendments to the legislation became apparent for a number of reasons. As one MEP involved in scrutinising the TPD legislation commented:

> So most times when I get a lobby from a company, they write to you [...]. They send me their amendment and, say, write me a letter and I can see where they come from and [what] they want to know. The tobacco industry had amendments only on paper, which they gave to MEPs. They didn't actually circulate them via e-mail. [...] So the key people who were working on the Directive, let's say [...], the rapporteur [...] shadow rapporteur [...] most of them were not given these amendments. They were only given to other people, because they thought that if they gave them to people, they would spot [...] that they were all saying... [the same]. When you see – you know, I've done a lot of laws in Europe – when you see eighty amendments all identical ... and they were pretty transparent, because most of their amendments were around packaging.

In keeping with TTC strategy, there were a high number of amendments tabled on the Directive at the committee stage. However, despite an extremely high volume of amendments, the progress of the Directive was not waylaid. As one member of the ENVI committee commented:

> And we had a vote in committee – there were thousands of amendments – and they hoped a thousand amendments would make it difficult. But if

> you know what you're doing, it's not. [...We] just drafted compromises, got them agreed and in the end we voted in an hour in the committee. So in one hour we finished the vote on tobacco products.

The industry demonstrated a nuanced understanding of how the internal organisation of the party groups functions in the EP and their ability to shape the position of even the larger parliamentary blocks by targeting a few key individuals amenable to their position. According to one policy actor with knowledge of the passage of the Directive in the EP, the industry sought to influence the position of the EPP to water down the EP position on labelling and to prevent the Directive moving out of the committee stage and onto the plenary:

> One, they were trying to reduce the size of the warnings on the packages to about fifty percent and, two, they were trying to prevent Linda McAvan from having a mandate to enter negotiations with the Commission which would've killed the Directive. [...] [The EPP] had agreed... their formal position was to vote in favour of reducing the size of the warnings to fifty percent. But that was by sleight of hand, they were deceived by the tobacco industry. What happens is the MEPs [in each party grouping] meet up [...] to decide their formal positions on each of the amendments. The attendance is very, very poor so what the industry did was they got all the MEPs who they had worried about jobs or they had supporting them for whatever reason, to turn up at that meeting. [...]. So they get all the MEPs who are... who they know are supportive of their views to turn up at that. Turnout is always very low at these things, but they had a majority in the room. Then when it goes to the Parliament, the MEPs don't actually know what they're voting for, and they're told 'how do you vote for Amendment 171 for European Tobacco Products Directive' and they see a little sign saying the formal EPP position. So it was all set up that the European Parliament would vote for... to reduce the size of the warnings to fifty percent.

The realisation of what had happened in the EPP group led to outcry from policy makers involved in the passage of the TPD, including rapporteur Linda McAvan and Irish Health Minister James Riley, who held the rotating presidency of the Council at the time, and whose party is itself a member of the EPP grouping. The respondent continued:

> What happened then was really interesting because you do realise what happened, they had their own rapporteur and he sent out correspondence to the EPP to say vote against our formal position which is unheard of in European

politics. So the EPP had their own rapporteur who pushed the formal EPP position. He just abandoned the post, he said this is crazy, and went against the former EPP position.

Once the legislation moved out of the committee stage, industry strategy shifted from potential amendment to seeking to delay agreement on the EP position in the EP Plenary:

It was always scheduled that we'd vote [in committee] in July and it would go to Plenary in September for the vote […]. And that was plenty of time, really; there was a holiday in between, but there was no difference between that and any other law. There was no rush to get it through the Plenary, it was a normal framework for those. […] And then they managed to persuade people in September, when we came out from the summer – they spent a lot of time in the summer persuading people – to delay the vote in the full Parliament. Because of course, by then you get to the end of 2013.

Here, the logic of the industry strategy to delay the progress of the TPD within the context of the electoral cycle of the EP is evident. In the end, the EP Plenary voted on the proposed text of the TPD in October 2013.

The success of the TTCs in marshalling support for their positions in the key EP committees, and proposing amendments, was echoed by other respondents. The industry again demonstrated their understanding of the institutional dynamic in play in the EP and the ability of committees other than ENVI, which may be more amenable to their arguments, to influence the content of the Directive. As this representative of a public health NGO which monitored the TPD negotiations commented:

There was a first phase where I think that things were going quite well for the tobacco industry, where they were able to mobilise a lot of allies in the European Parliament, in several key committees. Not the Environment Committee but the Internal Market and Trade Committee, for example, the votes were very beneficial for the tobacco industry, and you could really see that they had succeeded in mobilising allies there, which was also the strategy. But then also a backlash that then removed some of those gains that it looked like they were about to get. […] And particularly after the leak … of parts of their lobbying strategy, which then stiffened the resolve of a lot of pro-public health MEPs, but also broader than that, MEPs that felt that it was … it would be a disaster for the Parliament's reputation if it was seen to give into tobacco industry lobbying to the extent that it was starting to look like in some of the committees. And of course with the documents that revealed all

> the number of meetings that had happened and so on. And then the fact that the European Parliament elections were just around the corner also was an important factor. So that then meant that the pendulum swung back a bit.

According to one MEP involved in the TPD negotiations, it was noteworthy that fewer MEPs from the main political groupings (The EPP, the Progressive Alliance of Socialists and Democrats [S&D], and the Alliance of Liberals and Democrats for Europe [ALDE]) were willing to put forward amendments proposed by the tobacco industry than had been the case on previous tobacco legislation. The industry was thus much more reliant on members from the fringe political groupings which—because of the important yet often under-appreciated role played by political groupings in the EP—undermined the ability of TTCs to affect the debate:

> The problem they had was, they mainly had fringe politicians; they had no sense – if you're a lobbyist [...] if you pick a load of non-attached members ... UKIP [UK Independence Party] people ... to put amendments down for you, nobody from the main political groups will ... then you know that you're on the road to nowhere, really. And I mean, it's interesting, that's all they could get and that's what was good in the end. They got some mainstream EPP to put down the amendments for them, but not many. Not many would put them down.

Despite this, the TTCs were nevertheless able to get some centre-right MEPs to act for them, particularly those with strong free market or libertarian positions and other members of the centre-right EPP grouping from countries with weaker records on tobacco control and greater openness to direct engagement with the tobacco industry, such as Germany. According to another NGO actor, it was German EPP MEPs who were the pivotal actors in delaying the crucial vote in the plenary:

> What happened was the plenary vote was scheduled in September, and as a result of another Germany EPP intervention – the Germany EPP was dead against this Directive. As a result of a mobilisation by a number of those MEPs, the vote was postponed to October. You see, that was still the delay tactic.

The industry strategy of targeting the largest party block in the EP, the EPP, made sense in terms of the ideological leaning of this grouping (i.e. centre-right and pro-business). Within this grouping, Germany, as the most populous member state, has the largest number of MEPs, making these an obvious target in terms of simple arithmetic. However, there are other factors which explain the targeting of German delegates. First, German parliamentarians have a specific conception of the independence of the parliamentary mandate—which is sometimes juxtaposed to the Anglo-Saxon approach—which means MEPs are less reticent to meet with industry actors, or less willing to exclude certain groups from access. Second, Germany has a weak record on tobacco control and thus a political culture less antithetic to the tobacco industry, which retains significant economic interests and political connections. MEPs with industry holdings within their territories can be used by the industry to oppose unfavoured proposals in the EP and were used to lobby their colleagues who may support such measures. One German EPP MEP recounted to us that they had been strongly reprimanded by colleagues in their own national party grouping, particularly those with tobacco industry interests in their constituencies, for supporting measures opposed by the industry.

Whilst the EPP block was crucial, the targeting of German delegates by the industry extended beyond the more general overtures to the EPP. As the NGO respondent continues:

> And, again, you look at liberals from certain countries rather than others, the liberal group, the German Liberal Group in the old Parliament was quite large compared to now where they have almost nothing. Then they had eleven, thirteen, fifteen people, so it was quite large. But, you know, between the German EPP and then the German liberals, you had all of a sudden sixty votes. That's ten percent of the Parliament.

Delegates from other countries with close strategic relationships to the tobacco industry were targeted in similar ways. Asked if Germany was the main target of TTC lobbying, the respondent continued:

> I would say so, but the Spanish were also targeted. Spain is a main tobacco-growing country. Poland, Poland was there, well, the Polish MEPs were terrible in this respect. Again, a huge growing country. Bulgaria and Romania, for the same reason. The Czech Republic is because the Czech Republic is traditionally friendly. But, you know, if you add these up, all of a sudden you end up with 120–150 MEPs and that's a big group.

Alongside the ideological and national components of the industry strategy, there is an important temporal dimension which should be highlighted. Lobbying of the key institutions does not appear to have been completely sequential and the decision to target MEPs was taken in advance even of the publication of the Commission's initial draft Directive. Thus, whilst the industry was seeking to delay and water down the Commission proposals at the pre-proposal stage, they were already laying the groundwork for opposing its passage through the Parliament. As one MEP recounted:

> But, before the proposal was tabled, already there, the tobacco industry was quite active. The snus companies started already, I suppose, in 2009, to lobby and come around and talk to us.

Asked to clarify if they meant the lobbying in the EP began even before a concrete proposal for the Directive had been put forward by the Commission, they continued:

> Yeah. Quite some time before it, in fact. So, I saw a paper, I don't know who made it, but I got the impression that the tobacco industry had, more or less, talked to one third of all the members before the proposal was tabled. I don't know if that's true, but I got the impression anyway they were here and they also tried to get into contact with me.

In summary, the TTC strategy in the Parliament was, as across the EU institutions, to amend and delay the progress of the Directive, and focused to a large degree on the packaging proposals as a key issue to dilute. The industry again tailored their tactics to the dynamics and timetables of the specific institution. As with their targeting of various DGs in the Commission, the TTCs identified parliamentary committees outside of health which may be more amenable to their interests. Through their individual-level profiling of MEPs, they sought actors to table amendments for them and voice their objections to the Directive. They focused on party blocks ideologically less inclined to support regulation and more inclined to be pro-business (the EPP) and delegates from member states with weak approaches to tobacco control (e.g. Germany) and with tobacco industry presence. MEPs with individual, local connections to the industry were especially targeted. The industry was ubiquitous in its attempts to create opposition to the Directive in the EP at all stages of the process. Lobbying of MEPs began even before the publication of the Commission proposal and continued throughout.

However, as with the 'Dalligate' scandal, the political controversy which followed the leak of the PMI lobbying strategy undermined the industry's ability to engage MEPs.

Third-Party Lobbying

Demonstrating an awareness of the controversial nature of their industry, the TTCs' strategy in opposing the TPD was to work through third-party actors to a significant extent. This included the use of political consultancies, lobbying firms and public relations (PR) agencies in ways common to many commercial and non-commercial policy actors. However, it involved also the engagement, and formation of alliances with, other, more legitimately viewed, policy actors who had a plausible interest in the various aspects of the TPD under negotiation. According to one member of the ENVI committee, the use of proxies by the industry was vital to their strategy and meant they were not always visible to MEPs themselves. Unsurprisingly, the industry made use of political consultancies and lobbying firms to engage key policy actors, but also made use of law firms retained to represent their interests as conduits for their messaging on the TPD.

According to one EU civil servant with extensive knowledge of Brussels lobbying, this had emerged as an increasingly important lobbying tactic with the expanding presence of American law firms in Brussels, which brought with them influencing strategies developed in Washington. This was a potentially effective tactic for a number of reasons. Firstly, the very nature of the EU system means that lawyers play a central role and connections between officials and law firms are necessarily extensive. As one official stated:

> Also the European Union system is extremely legalistic. The lawyers are crucial, so in every way and sense … lawyers inside the institutions, outside the institutions, we do a lot in revolving doors, so you see a lot of lobby firms hire the tough lawyers from the Commission, etc.

Law firms are also subject to client privilege arrangements, undermining the possibility that they may be called on to disclose who their clients are; they are not officially lobbyists, so will not be listed on registers of lobbyists, and they represent a number of clients. For all these reasons, it may be unclear to policy-makers that they are in fact engaging with tobacco industry agents. At the very least, politicians who are reticent about being seen to meet with tobacco interests may nonetheless be prepared to meet with law firms. Consequently, operating through these intermediaries offers TTCs considerable advantages. As one EU civil servant commented when asked who the main actors were representing the tobacco industry in Brussels:

> Well I don't know. And this is one of the problems; you don't know. Unless you get financial transparency you don't know, but you have suspicions. And the industry's got third parties as they call them. Third parties, definitely they work through a lot of law firms. And again, the Commission would say […] "Oh, our legal services meeting with law firms is a legal meeting, not a lobby meeting". Of course a good lobbyist would blur the lines. They get in the door on a legal issue and then they go, "Oh well" - and you can discuss law in lots of ways and the use of law. But law firms, PR firms yeah, absolutely.

Transparency issues were also a key concern when dealing with third-party actors, such as law firms and PR consultancies, representing industry interests:

> But again there's no transparency in some PR firms, so you don't know. So often it's suspicious. And then again, from my experience, front groups they have –in terms of organisations they have generic-sounding names, you know? Europeans for a Future Dynamic European Economy of…. some generic-sounding names, very little information on their website about who really they are, no financial information. But then great access. You often see them having – they have Commissioners, they have judges, they have brilliant people coming to their events. Why do they have such amazing access? […] So it's hard – unless you see the financial information it's very hard to see who they really are.

An MEP who was engaged with the debates around the TPD, was initially unaware of the connection between law firms requesting meetings on legal issues relating to TPD and the tobacco industry:

> You know, the law firms they do it when it comes to copyright, IP [intellectual property] questions, they do it a lot in that. In the beginning, I took a lot of meetings because I thought, "Oh, well". Being a rep [MEP] you didn't know anything about it. But then I realised later on that they were, in fact, lobbyists, so now I'm more, you know, kind of, "Well, do I have an interest in having a meeting with them?" If yes, then okay, if not, then no, thank you, because they're a lobbyist.

In addition to the use of consultancies and law firms, TTCs sought to highlight the economic effects of the TPD, focusing on the issue of employment. They often focused on MEPs with tobacco manufacturing or ancillary facilities in their constituencies and used this as a pretext for seeking engagement on the TPD. As one MEP commented:

> What they did try was get the packaging industry up in arms. They were going to lose all their jobs, so what they did, they would.... [A city in my region], for example, had a big cigarette packaging company and so they tried to get constituency-based packaging companies, or locally based to lobby individual MEPs, and so they would ask for meetings.

This was mirrored by the experience of another MEP from a different member state and her colleagues in the same national and party grouping:

> So, they contacted him and his staff and then they went to my staff, trying to put pressure on me. [...] Yeah, and saying that, "Well, we have this and it's all in his constituency and you need to take care of this. And the trade unions are putting pressure on us". So, they knew that they did not really succeed in doing it directly to me, but they tried via other colleagues to do it.

The tobacco industry also sought to engage other, less controversial, sectors and industries that may have been adversely affected by issues in the TPD, attempting to find common purpose with them. In particular, TTCs sought to engage retailers who may be prepared to speak out on the issue of standardised packaging. As one MEP engaged in the TPD debates commented:

> The other proxy was retailers, and they tried to recruit small businesses, retailers. So I'd get phone calls – and you know, this guy keeps phoning my office and it was Easter holiday [...]. And he was saying things like well, she ought to be in her constituency, I want to see her and all this, because I represent local shopkeepers and they want to see her. [...] Anyway, my office got a bit fed-up with this guy, so you know, "who are you?". You know, [...] he worked for British American Tobacco, he wasn't a small retailer, he was a consultant who was being paid to organise British small retailers. So they did have – just as they've got Forest, which is the consumers, they've got a small retailer group, who was funded by the tobacco industry. And what they were doing, they were again, through constituency contacts saying I'm a [local] corner shop and I want to meet you. Because that makes it

> more difficult to say no, doesn't it, than saying I'm not going to meet Philip Morris or British American Tobacco […], but I'm a corner shop from your constituency. But they weren't really corner shops; behind them all were paid lobbyists of tobacco – everywhere you were, everywhere you'd look, underneath it all were the paid lobbyists for the tobacco industry.

This quote reveals not just the use made of the retail sector but also the use of local actors to engage participants in the debate. This strategy is particularly effective when targeting MEPs, given the connections with the specific areas they serve and their responsibility to represent the interests of their constituents. This is particularly the case for local shopkeepers and newsagents who are often at the heart of local communities and who may be afforded more sympathy than large-scale retailers if it appears their livelihoods are at risk. Industry actors also used any industry presence in MEPs' local constituencies to open lines of communication with MEPs, which, in some instances, proved a successful means of influencing the content of the Directive. As an EU civil servant commented:

> If you look back at the amendments on the Tobacco Directive there was some Irish MEPs who made them, which could be seen as pro-tobacco industry amendments. And I think the way that happened was it had this – like they do all over Europe – there was a small factory in the middle of Ireland and made these little bags for – and one of the directives was to change the size of the bags, I don't know, of the tobacco. And of course they got the local company to go on to local radio, saying that this was going to destroy a hundred or two hundred jobs or whatever.

The respondent continued that meetings would often be presented as being highly circumscribed and being limited to specific, often technical, issues. Whilst this appeared to offer more legitimate grounds to meet with the industry, it could also serve as a pretext for wider-ranging discussions of more obvious political importance to the industry:

> And of course local MEPs who care about their constituents will obviously try to – while they say, "Well, we're not in favour of tobacco", this technical thing about a technical – you know, because machinery is not changed and – you know, they would've maybe not seen the dangers of these amendments. It wasn't just amendments on the size for the machinery, it was actually then twenty other amendments thrown in because the lobby – whoever the lobby or middleman they were talking to – used that opening to a very local

> issue to add in more amendments. So that kind of tactic probably would be used all – I'm very sure they use it all over Europe. They know exactly how to appeal to that local politician, and every politician will listen to their constituency. And then once you open up a channel of communication, then because most MEPs are not aware of the issues, and if you're not following the issues, a lot of issues are very technical. And then before you know it a lot of amendments come in. And if you get amendments coming in from different parts of Europe and different political groups, then it has a much better chance of passing.

Even where the contacts are not linked to an MEP's specific local constituency, attempts to engage them would be channelled through contacts in their own country or region. As one Danish MEP commented:

> Yeah, they contacted me through Danish people. They requested a meeting and I said yes to that meeting. We had it in the Members' … not the Members' Bar, the Tractor Bar, in public so to speak. They tried to talk to me and tried to come into me about their problems on the packaging issues, labelling issues. And I didn't agree with them and I discussed with them and afterwards they came back to me by email trying to, you know, argue further on. And they also kept on having a dialogue with my assistant at that time, because I said I don't want to discuss with them any longer. I'd given them this one meeting and then we had … But also, some other tobacco manufacturers in Denmark, not the cigarettes but the pipe tobacco, they had a lot of issues on … and snus, they had a lot of issues on the packaging in general and also the substances, the ban on certain substances.

The two preceding quotes also demonstrate the dangers for MEPs in engaging with industry actors or their proxies on any issue at all. Once lines of communication are established, they appear to use this as the basis to further develop the relationship, either by moving the conversation on to new issues outside the remit of the agreed meeting or to use this as a pretext for further dialogue and on-going communication.

On other occasions, the concept of local lobbying took on another dimension, with local actors such as small business operators contacting MEPs at their constituency homes. As the assistant of one MEP commented:

> He received, in his private letterbox of his house, his home, a sort of alarm letter by his local newspaper dealer, who is obviously also a tobacco seller. This particular person addressed him personally as someone who is also a customer

> and saying, "Listen, you are a Member of Parliament, you are dealing with TPD. I am very worried because if certain proposals would be accepted by the European Parliament this would be disastrous for my business". It was a bit remarkable. Most lobby letters you receive are either by lobby groups or [interest] groups, NGOs, company umbrella groups or if they're big companies they can afford to have this kind of a lobby work, PR work themselves. One particular newspaper shop owner sending this letter which was obviously very well formulated, very well argumented (sic) and with knowledge behind on a very timely moment – I mean well in advance. Later on we found out that there were more MEPs receiving such letters and it was orchestrated – it was organised by – now I have to think very well, there was an umbrella organisation in [our country] that basically did it on the [country-wide] scale but I think, if I'm not mistaken, MEPs from other countries also received similar letters. So, it was centrally driven by umbrella lobby organisations on a national level.

The messaging and the channels through which MEPs were contacted were tailored not just to their nationality or the cities and regions from which they came but also to their political ideologies. This meant framing arguments in terms of issues to which they were more likely to be sympathetic and through channels allied to the political movements of which they were part. For example, trade unions were used to engage MEPs in the left-of-centre S&D group. As an S&D MEP recounted:

> The trade unions I should have mentioned as well, of course. They tried to get the trade unions on board – well they did. [A specific trade union] came to lobby me, and they recruited … they recruited former colleagues of mine to work for them.

In addition, the respondent felt it was clear that the union's position statement on TPD had been strongly influenced by the industry:

> Oh yeah, it had been written by them, I think, because their officer didn't turn up. The official from [the union] didn't turn up with them and they had this very official-looking thing [document], which they didn't, you know … I mean, at the end of the day, here's people who work, it's very difficult; they're low-paid workers working, packing cigarettes, you know, and they've seen their industry has been decimated and it's lost market share, but they've off-shored it, because it's labour intensive; it's been off-shored more and more, this sort of work anyway.

The union in question asked the MEP if they would meet a delegation of workers from a factory in their home country. However, rather than meeting in their constituency office, they took a delegation of employees to Brussels:

> I met the workers from the factory who came with [the union], so they brought people from [a city in my constituency] to Brussels [...]. They didn't meet me as the industry; I went to meet some [union] delegation where there were workers from my constituency in that. I mean, I didn't know who I was going to meet; I just knew I was meeting [the] union.

The industry thus clearly understood the issues around employment, which would be of concern to centre-left politicians and the potential dilemma they would face between their objectives of protecting the livelihoods of low-paid workers and the public health goals behind the TPD. Given these politicians' close association with the trade union movement, these were identified as a key conduit for industry messages, which were conveyed to MEPs at meetings not just with union officials but with the very workers who may be affected by any subsequent factory closures and who may be thought to constitute the natural electoral constituency for politicians on the left. This shows a keen sense of the psychological pressure which could be applied to MEPs by the industry, by identifying the most effective messengers for their position. The use of third-party lobbyists discussed in this section poses particular challenges to the effective implementation of Article 5.3 of the FCTC, especially in relation to the transparency of officials' and representatives' contacts with the industry, given that it may not be clear that such third parties are acting on behalf of the industry (Hawkins and Holden 2018).

Insider Lobbying

The use of national, local and ideological connections to participants was indicative of a wider use of direct political contacts including former politicians and people currently or previously active in political parties and movements connected to MEPs. One MEP recounted how they were lobbied by a prominent activist in their national party:

> The guy who called, I knew him from earlier, in the past he was working for some politicians in [my country] and he himself was a former Youth

> [member of my party]. So, I knew who he was and he's a well-known guy in [my country]. But, he presented himself as representing the industry. But, in a, "Hello, [...] how are you?" You know, things like that.

Issues also arose at the EU level because of the practice of allowing former MEPs to retain their security credentials after they leave office. With continued access to the EP, and political connections built up from their time in the assembly and in party machines, they are ideally placed to act as lobbyists and conduits for corporate arguments on future legislation. The MEP cited previously commented:

> But, of course, we're also, as a Parliament, pushing for this mandatory lobbyist register et cetera. And once it's there, I think that we should have a, kind of, a work saying that people that are not registered here in the Parliament should not be allowed access to the Parliament. And we could do more also for former members of the Parliament, as you know, we have this badge for coming into the house, even when you are a former member you have a badge, you can come and go whenever you want to. You can blend. In Brussels airport, if there is a car picking up some MEPs and there are seats left over, you can go as a former MEP coming into the house. Even though you're working for a company, you're allowed to go around, all around in the Parliament. And I saw former colleagues doing that and they were working for the tobacco industry.

For this respondent the blurred lines which exist between current and former MEPs drifting in and out of the EP facilities, and using EP services, has the consequence of also blurring the lines between legislators and lobbyists in the EP. According to the same MEP, this makes current members more susceptible to lobbying:

> So they came here, you know, as a former colleague saying, "Hello, how are you?" et cetera, and then, suddenly I had to remember, "Oh, is it a colleague or is it a lobbyist?" So, here, I also think that we could do more. Even though we have, as I heard it, we have rules in place saying that you're not allowed to use your badge if you're coming here as a lobbyist, more or less. But, in fact, it is what is happening.

Another MEP involved in the TPD process also highlighted how a former colleague from the EP had approached her, revealing that they were working for a branch of the tobacco industry, and she had declined to discuss the issue of the TPD with them. The respondent was aware also of other colleagues who had been approached by the industry also. The issue of former MEPs being able to lobby on behalf of private sector actors, including the tobacco industry, is just one example of the wider connections that exist between political actors within the EU, which is explored in the following section.

EU Officials and TTCs

The connections between the tobacco industry and officials in the EU institutions has been widely discussed, particularly in relation to the Dalligate scandal (Peeters et al. 2015; Costa et al. 2014; Berteletti et al. 2017). This extended to the role played by the most senior officials in the Commission and their handling of the Dalli case. In addition, questions have been raised about the 'revolving door' of political appointments in which former officials assume lucrative roles in the private sector whilst retaining significant contacts within the machinery of the institutions. One example of this is the case of Michel Petite, the former Director-General of the European Commission Legal Services and Head of Cabinet to former Commission President Romano Prodi, who has since gone on to work for the law firm Clifford Chance in the area of 'government relations and public policy' (Tobacco Tactics 2016e). Clifford Chance not only has tobacco industry clients, including Philip Morris, it has failed to sign up to the EU's transparency register (Tobacco Tactics 2016f). Petite has extensive experience of tobacco-control issues within the Commission, including negotiating an anti-contraband and counterfeiting deal with PMI on behalf of the Commission in 2004. Since moving to Clifford Chance, Petite has reportedly represented Philip Morris and brokered meetings between Commission officials and the tobacco industry (Peeters et al. 2015; Tobacco Tactics 2016e). Nevertheless, Petite was appointed Chairman of the Commission's ad hoc Ethical Committee, in which his remit included overseeing potential conflicts of interest within the Commission (Tobacco Tactics 2016e).

The case of Michel Petite was raised repeatedly by interview respondents as an example of the potential for conflicts of interest in the EU and the Commission's contacts with the tobacco industry. However, this was not an isolated example. One respondent highlighted the case of Klaus-Heiner Lehne, a former German MEP and Germany's Auditor at the European Court of Auditors. Since 2003 Lehne has been a partner in a German law firm, Taylor Wessing, which includes Japan Tobacco International (JTI) amongst its clients (Tobacco Tactics 2016g; Rivasi 2013). This led fellow MEP, Michèle Rivasi, to seek clarification from Lehne about his firm's involvement with the industry. While Lehne denied there was a conflict of interest, he did not deny tobacco industry connections and stated it his responsibility to meet with all relevant stakeholders on issues in order to form balanced opinions. Lehne was Chair of the EP Committee on Legal Affairs (JURI) during the TPD process and was identified as a high-priority lobbying target in the leaked PMI strategy documents, given his positions on key components of the Directive (Tobacco Tactics 2016g). The interview respondent noted that JURI's legal opinion on the TPD opposed certain aspects of the Commission's draft, such as the proposal that warning labels cover 75% of the packet, concluding instead that they should be limited to just 50% (European Parliament Committee on Legal Affairs 2013).

It is possible that connections between the industry and EU-level policy actors may have been a means for them to collect important information about the legislative timetable and the very latest content of proposals. Leaked PMI strategy documents show a high level of information on the progress of the legislation, including the dates of proposed meetings, hearings and votes which would have been crucial in planning and executing their influencing strategy. On some occasions it seems they were able to get information ahead even of elected members of the EP and their officials. As one MEP recounted:

> One thing I was quite surprised by, was the fact that [...] during the trialogue, in the end, sometimes I got information from the tobacco industry about the content of the negotiations before I got information from colleagues [...]. And, not me directly, because I said, "I don't want", but one of my colleagues.

Summary

The tobacco industry was able to exercise significant influence over the development of the TPD. Whilst proposals to introduce SP at the EU level were mooted in initial proposals for the revised Directive, these were removed at the very earliest stages of the policy process, before a formal proposal emanated from the Commission. This may reflect the ability of industry actors to engage with key policy actors, including those at the very highest levels of the Commission. It reflects also the wider assumptions which underpin Commission activities and the on-going inertia in the development of tobacco-control debates at the EU level, which continue to balance corporate interests against those of public health. This is evident in the inadequate steps taken by the EU institutions to implement Article 5.3 of the FCTC (Hawkins and Holden 2018). It demonstrates also the effectiveness of engaging with policy developments at the earliest possible stage in order to circumscribe the parameters of political debate and 'anchor' subsequent developments to this initial proposal. This is a particularly effective tactic in EU policy development, in which legislation can only be enacted on the basis of Commission proposals and where there is significant path dependency once draft legislation emerges. However, TTCs were influential at all stages of the policy process, tailoring their approach to the different institutions and phases of the process. Whilst industry actors failed to prevent the adoption of a revised TPD, they were able to delay its enactment and implementation, prevent the adoption of SP at the EU level and water down increased labelling requirements (Peeters et al. 2015; Costa et al. 2014; Berteletti et al. 2017). However, the Directive included explicit recognition that member states could go beyond what were identified as minimum packaging requirements and so ban colour branding and implement SP. The battle for SP in Europe thus moved to the national level.

Bibliography

Bachrach, P., & Baratz, M. S. (1962). Two faces of power. *The American Political Science Review, 56*(4), 947–952.

Berteletti, F., King, J., Burch, J., & Friedlander, A. T. (2017). Campaign for a revised Tobacco Products Directive in the European Union: Lessons learnt. *Tobacco Control, 26*, 464–467.

Costa, H., Gilmore, A. B., Peeters, S., McKee, M., & Stuckler, D. (2014). Quantifying the influence of the tobacco industry on EU governance: Automated content analysis of the EU Tobacco Products Directive. *Tobacco Control, 23*, 473–478.

European Ombudsman. (2016). *Decision concerning the European Commission's compliance with the Tobacco Control Convention (852/2014/LP)*. Brussels: European Ombudsman. Available at https://www.ombudsman.europa.eu/en/decision/en/73774. Accessed 28 February 2019.

European Parliament Committee on Legal Affairs. (2013). *Draft opinion of the Committee on Legal Affairs for the Committee on the Environment, Public Health and Food Safety* (2012/0366[COD]). Available at http://www.europarl.europa.eu/sides/getDoc.do?pubRef=-%2f%2fEP%2f%2fNONSGML%2bCOMPARL%2bPE-510.591%2b01%2bDOC%2bPDF%2bV0%2f%2fEN. Accessed 1 March 2019.

Hawkins, B., & Holden, C. (2018). European Union implementation of Article 5.3 of the Framework Convention of Tobacco Control. *Globalization and Health, 14,* 79.

Hörz, M. (2014). *Looking back at the tobacco lobbying battle: Philip Morris' allies in the European Parliament.* Corporate Europe Observatory. Available at https://corporateeurope.org/power-lobbies/2014/05/looking-back-tobacco-lobbying-battle-philip-morris-allies-european-parliament. Accessed 1 March 2019.

Lukes, S. (1974). *Power: A radical view.* London and New York: Macmillan.

MacKenzie, R., Mathers, A., Hawkins, B., Eckhardt, J., & Smith, J. (2018). The tobacco industry's challenge to standardised packaging: A comparative analysis of issue framing in public relations campaigns in four countries. *Health Policy, 122*(9), 1001–1011.

Peeters, S., Costa, H., Stuckler, D., McKee, M., & Gilmore, A. B. (2015). The revision of the 2014 European Tobacco Products Directive: An analysis of the tobacco industry's attempts to 'break the health silo'. *Tobacco Control.* https://doi.org/10.1136/tobaccocontrol-2014-051919.

Rivasi, M. (2013). *Directive Tabac: Lettre à Klaus-Heiner Lehne, Eurodéputé (Group PPE) Rapporteur du Texte en Commission Juri.* Available at http://www.michele-rivasi.eu/au-parlement/directive-tabac-lettre-a-klaus-heiner-lehne-eurodepute-groupe-ppe-rapporteur-du-texte-en-commission-juri/. Accessed 1 March 2019.

Smith, K. E., Fooks, H., Collin, J., Weishaar, H., Mandal, S. & Gilmore, A. B. (2010). 'Working the system'—British American Tobacco's influence on the European Union Treaty and its implications for policy: An analysis of internal tobacco industry documents. *PLoS Medicine, 7*(1), e1000202.

Tobacco Tactics. (2016a). *TPD: Delaying the process of consultation.* Tobacco Tactics. Available at http://tobaccotactics.org/index.php/TPD:_Delaying_the_Process_of_Consultation. Accessed 1 March 2019.

Tobacco Tactics. (2016b). *TPD: Dalligate.* Tobacco Tactics. Available at http://www.tobaccotactics.org/index.php?title=TPD:_Dalligate. Accessed 1 March 2019.

Tobacco Tactics. (2016c). *PMI's lobbying campaign to undermine the TPD.* Tobacco Tactics. Available at http://tobaccotactics.org/index.php/PMI%E2%80%99s_Lobbying_Campaign_to_Undermine_the_TPD. Accessed 1 March 2019.

Tobacco Tactics. (2016d). *Third party techniques*. Tobacco Tactics. Available at http://www.tobaccotactics.org/index.php/Third_Party_Techniques. Accessed 1 March 2019.

Tobacco Tactics. (2016e). *Michel Petite*. Tobacco Tactics. Available at http://www.tobaccotactics.org/index.php?title=Michel_Petite. Accessed 1 March 2019.

Tobacco Tactics. (2016f). *Clifford Chance*. Tobacco Tactics. Available at http://www.tobaccotactics.org/index.php?title=Clifford_Chance. Accessed 1 March 2019.

Tobacco Tactics. (2016g). *Klaus-Heiner Lehne*. Tobacco Tactics. Available at http://www.tobaccotactics.org/index.php/Klaus-Heiner_Lehne. Accessed 1 March 2019.

CHAPTER 4

The Member-State Level: Standardised Packaging in Ireland and Beyond

Abstract This chapter presents the study's findings in relation to the development of standardised cigarette packaging in Ireland. Ireland was the first European Union (EU) member state to introduce standardised packaging (SP) laws, closely followed by the UK. The findings demonstrate that transnational tobacco companies (TTCs) allocated considerable resources in an attempt to block the introduction of SP in Ireland, fearing that successful adoption in that country would lead other EU member states to follow suit. TTCs mobilised a range of third-party actors to attempt to block SP in Ireland. TTCs' tactics in this case are consistent with the existence of broader, globally coordinated TTC strategies to resist the adoption of strengthened tobacco packaging laws across a range of jurisdictions.

Keywords Standardised packaging · Plain packaging · EU Tobacco Products Directive · Ireland · European Union · Transnational tobacco companies

The events at the EU level were crucial for developments in tobacco-control policy at the national level, and particularly the plans by some member states to introduce standardised packaging (SP). Whilst, as detailed in the previous chapter, a commitment to introduce such a measure Europe-wide was absent from the Commission's draft legislation, the Directive did include a

B. Hawkins et al., *The Battle for Standardised Cigarette Packaging in Europe*, Palgrave Studies in Public Health Policy Research,
https://doi.org/10.1007/978-3-030-31034-9_4

specific acknowledgement that member states could go beyond the packaging requirements in the TPD, which were to be viewed as a minimum requirement only. Interview respondents in Brussels and Dublin agreed that the inclusion of this clause was vital to the success of national campaigns on SP. One respondent claimed that it provided 'air cover' for the national campaign, providing an explicit rationale for the policy, enshrined in EU law. It was hoped also that this would shield governments from legal action by the TTCs at the EU level. As will be discussed below, this was not the case in Ireland, but the explicit inclusion of the acceptability of SP in the TPD was crucial in defending cases that were brought by the tobacco industry.

The Irish government announced its intention to become only the second country in the world to introduce SP in May 2013. The announcement came as the Taoiseach (Irish Prime Minister) and other senior ministers were being heavily criticised for meeting with a tobacco industry delegation (Beesley 2013a). Six American business groups (including the US Chamber of Commerce) quickly reacted to the announcement, urging the Irish Government to rethink the proposals. Despite this, Cabinet approved the General Scheme of the Public Health (Standardised Packaging of Tobacco) Bill in November 2013, and a Joint Oireachtas (Irish Parliament) Committee on Health and Children was invited to undertake a consultation on the proposals. In March 2014, an independent review of the evidence was published (Hammond 2014), which concluded that SP would have a positive impact on Ireland's public health goals. This was followed in April by the Joint Oireachtas Committee's report, which also strongly supported the introduction of SP. Throughout this period, TTCs and associated actors campaigned extensively to prevent the Bill being introduced, flooding the Oireachtas consultation with responses and undertaking aggressive media campaigns such as 'Plain packs plain stupid' to discredit the policy and the evidence underpinning it (Hawkins et al. 2018). Despite this onslaught, the Bill was introduced in the Irish Parliament in June 2014 and was adopted into law in May 2015.

The debates around SP must be viewed in light of the prevailing political and economic conditions in Ireland at the time of the proposal's development. Ireland had been widely praised by actors in the field of tobacco control and public health for the leadership it had shown in becoming the first EU member state to introduce a ban on smoking in public places in March 2004. This proved to be a catalyst for similar measures elsewhere in the EU, including the UK. The experience of the smoking ban, and the actions of the tobacco industry in opposing this, had a profound effect on public perceptions about the right of governments to regulate to protect public health and the legitimacy of TTCs as policy actors. Whilst governments' right to regulate dangerous products to protect public health is widely accepted, the credibility of the tobacco industry has been undermined. For the public health community, the experience of the smoking ban cemented the idea that a small country such as Ireland can act as a policy entrepreneur within the EU, developing new areas of public policy even in the face of significant opposition by powerful economic actors. For those in the tobacco industry, and other opponents of public health regulations, it demonstrated the capacity for 'policy contagion' between countries in Europe and between the member-state and the European levels. Policy developments, even in small member states, had the capacity to lead to fundamental changes in regulation and culture across the EU.

Between the introduction of the smoking ban in 2004 and the announcement of the SP measures by Health Minister James Reilly in May 2013, Ireland had experienced an economic shock of unprecedented magnitude in the history of the country since independence. In the preceding decades, Ireland had experienced a period of significant economic growth, driven largely by foreign direct investment (FDI) from the US and facilitated through further investment and infrastructure spending via the EU structural development programmes, following Ireland's entry to the then European Economic Community (EEC) in 1973. Ireland's economic model was of an open economy encouraging investment through low levels of corporation tax and a flexible and increasingly skilled labour market within the European single market. This had led to an unprecedented economic boom but had also left its economy, and the banking system in particular, highly exposed to the vagaries of the global economy. One respondent who followed policy debates around SP in Dublin and Brussels went as far as to claim that the scale of the economic challenges faced by Ireland at the time were so severe that they represented an existential threat to the Republic:

> I think [...] you've got to realise that this is a pro-business country, which is now in recovery, but which was in the depths of a huge financial crisis. One of the worst bank collapses in the western world. The worst crisis to face this state since the Second World War when the state is neutral right? And one in which the very survival of the state is in question. And all of this

> took place at a time when government was really keen to maintain its pro-business credentials. And it took place at a time when the Irish government had come under great pressure from its European partners to increase the rate of corporate tax.

As the consequences of the global financial crisis played out, Ireland was forced to seek a bailout of its banks from the European Union institutions. In this context Ireland found itself under renewed pressure within the EU to alter its economic policies and, in particular, to raise its levels of corporation tax. These had been widely criticised by the European Commission and by other member states, including France and Germany, which feared the Irish model may lead to internal tax avoidance by corporations within the single market and a 'race to the bottom' amongst tax authorities, offering ever lower rates of tax in an effort to retain corporations domiciled within the territories. This historical context is of key importance in understanding the political strategy employed by the tobacco industry to oppose SP in Ireland.

Opposition at the EU Level

The Irish government was placed under significant pressure to reverse its decision to introduce SP from other member states at the EU level. These efforts came in the context not only of Ireland's shorter-term economic difficulties but longer-term debates within the EU about the economic policies pursued by the Irish government. More specifically, this centred on concern raised by the European Commission and other member states about Ireland's corporation tax regime, which was at the heart of its strategy to attract FDI. The previous respondent described the context of the discussion about SP at the EU level as:

> A situation in which both the current Taoiseach and his immediate predecessor were under pressure of European leaders from Nicolas Sarkozy and Angela Merkel, in a very, very overt way that Ireland must change its laws around corporate taxation. They came under huge pressure. And the government held firm. Reforms have been introduced in the intervening periods but, you know, in a scenario where the government was fighting to maintain its credentials and fighting to maintain the stability of the state and to rebuild its finances it seems to me there would have been some potency to whatever lobbying was going on.

Consequently, it was in the context of extreme economic and political pressure at the EU level—as a recipient of a bailout, compelled to expend significant amounts of political capital to defend its economic model—that the Irish government was forced to defend its proposed tobacco packaging measures. This afforded significant opportunities to policy actors opposed to SP to attempt to stymie the measures at the EU level, by articulating their narrow concerns about SP in relation to wider economic and political tensions at play and allying their interests to the specific policy agendas of other member states.

EU member states have a formal requirement to notify the Commission of proposed amendments to regulations and technical standards with potential implications for the functioning of the single market. This is followed by a three-month period in which member states may scrutinise and comment on proposals prior to their adoption. In cases in which there are potential implications for the free movement of goods or services, or other aspects of EU law, both the Commission and member states have the right to submit detailed opinions on the proposals during an additional three-month standstill for goods and one month for services. In the case of the Irish SP laws, opposition was raised by ten member states in total (Bulgaria, the Czech Republic, Greece, Hungary, Italy, Poland, Portugal, Romania, Slovakia and Spain), representing over half the population of the EU, which submitted detailed opinions to the Commission on the draft laws (European Commission 2014). This represented an unprecedented level of opposition for a piece of Irish legislation (O'Connor 2015). The notification process requires member states to take comments into account as far as possible in proceeding with the legislation, but falls short of affording other states an effective veto over domestic legislation. However, the consensus model of decision-making within the EU—even in areas where qualified majority voting is provided for—and the recognition of national governments that they may eventually find themselves on the other side of a debate, needing concessions from other member states in areas of acute national interest, creates strong incentives for governments to seek agreement for their policies. The degree of opposition to SP would have placed significant political pressure on Ireland to accommodate member states' objections. In the end, the Irish government did revise some details of its proposed legislation in light of the consultation, but maintained its commitment to the core elements of the policy.

Whilst the extent of the engagement, if any, between these member states and the tobacco industry is unclear, the arguments they used against the measures were closely aligned with those of the industry. A further respondent with knowledge of policy developments in Dublin and Brussels commented:

> The only country that came in, that wrote in in our favour was the UK. A few countries made no observations which is perfectly normal, some of these countries don't make observations on legislation. But I mean the arguments were straight out of the tobacco industry book, they were saying first we didn't have the authority to do this under the Tobacco Products Directive which it looks like it's going to be hard to get in the European Court of Justice. Secondly, they were talking about their intellectual property rights. You know, it's exactly the… it has similar elements to the tobacco industry line.

Whilst we cannot know in this instance whether national governments opposed to SP were representing concerns articulated to them by the industry, the recruitment of national governments to pursue their interests within intergovernmental institutions is an established tobacco industry tactic. Indeed, this approach has been deployed in the context of the WTO—in which only member states have legal standing to initiate disputes—to recruit compliant governments to oppose Australia's plain packaging measures (Eckhardt et al. 2016; Hawkins and Holden 2016).

The challenges to the SP measures were, however, not limited to other governments. MEPs opposed to SP also lobbied the Irish government and Taoiseach Enda Kenny (McEnroe 2014a, b). Similar concerns were also articulated by business associations from other EU member states, and some beyond the EU. As an NGO actor details:

> I have a list […] now these would've been companies and associations that would have sent letters to the, to the Irish Government […] it's the usual suspects there in terms of JTI [Japan Tobacco International] and European cigar manufacturers. But then you look further down the list and you see Tax Payers Association of Europe, the German Brand Association […], the US Chamber of Commerce of Mongolia, the US Taxpayers Protection Alliance and the Indonesian Farmers Association. Now one thing that at a European level that we, that became a bit of news here as well was the fact that there was a group of European People's Party, EPP members, who lobbied the Prime Minister here as well to say do not go ahead with plain packaging.

Cultural and Economic Ties with the US

The extent of American FDI in Ireland reflected the deep, long-standing cultural ties between Ireland and the US, forged through extensive emigrations from Ireland to the US and an Irish-American diaspora which maintains a clear identity and close emotional ties to their ancestral homeland. At no time is this more obvious than in the annual St Patrick's Day celebrations to commemorate Ireland's patron saint. The importance of St Patrick's Day in both Irish and American culture is symbolised by the tradition that the Irish Taoiseach spends St Patrick's Day not in Dublin but in Washington, DC, where he attends a series of functions, the pinnacle of which is a meeting with the President. As one respondent following policy developments in Dublin and Brussels commented:

> It is the practice in Dublin that an assortment of government ministers would travel around the world, around St. Patrick's Day, for official functions all over the world [...] and the practice for many years has been Taoiseach in Washington on St Patrick's Day and there's a ceremony at the White House every year, a shamrock ceremony at which the Taoiseach presents whoever is the American President with a bowl of shamrock. This is deeply engrained in Irish political culture that this takes place.

The annual visit by the Taoiseach presents organisations with interests in Ireland, including business associations, with the opportunity to engage with the Irish government at the highest possible level. One respondent with knowledge of the Taoiseach's 2014 itinerary highlights that the Chamber of Commerce were aware of the tobacco packaging issue prior to the meeting:

> On such occasions there would be other meetings which would take place in and around that ceremony and, you know, [...] immediately in advance of that particular visit last year, the first official event of the Taoiseach's visit to Washington on that occasion was a meeting in the US Chamber of Commerce and it was immediately prior to that that the US Chamber wrote to the Taoiseach, said we remain very concerned about this.

The importance of these trips by Irish politicians to the US as a lobbying opportunity for corporations with interests in Ireland was corroborated by an EU civil servant with contacts in Irish politics:

> I know on a personal basis, I know a former Irish – very senior Irish minister who said every time he went to America he was pulled aside by congressmen and senators about Ireland's position on tobacco. So that kind of influence, you know, you can't capture that anywhere. [...] You know, Irish ministers go for trade issues, for innovation issues, for St. Patrick's Day, lots of issues. But he said every time he went, no matter what the meeting was about, he would be pulled aside privately and always – especially obviously on the plain packaging issue in Ireland. So that kind of influence and that kind of influencing is extremely hard to capture.

These attempts to influence the Irish government were widely reported in the press at the time (Beesley 2014a). Interviewees with knowledge of the policy process also explained that there was a significant additional correspondence between business associations and the Irish government, outlining their reservations about the proposed introduction of SP. Further correspondence emanated from business organisations in the US including the US Chamber of Commerce. For example, the President and CEO of the Chamber, Tom Donohue, wrote to Taoiseach Enda Kenny reiterating concerns that SP laws would undermine intellectual property (IP) rights that had been raised at a meeting between the two at the US Chamber of Commerce the previous March. In addition, correspondence was sent to Kenny and the Irish Ambassador to the US, Anne Anderson, by a collection of business associations: The Emergency Committee for American Trade, The National Association of Manufacturers, The National Foreign Trade Council, The Transatlantic Business Council, The United States Council for International Business and the US Chamber of Commerce, raising concerns about the proposed tobacco packaging measures in light of the unresolved WTO case against similar measures in Australia (Beesley 2014b, c). The theme of the letters from the US was that there may be broader implications for Ireland in pursuing SP and that this may send an unwanted message to potential and actual foreign investors. Given the close economic relationship between the US and Ireland and the reliance of a significant segment of the Irish economy on US foreign direct investment, concerns of this nature being raised would have been treated with the utmost seriousness by the Irish Government.

The pro-tobacco stance taken by the Chamber would suggest a significant degree of influence by tobacco industry members over the activities of the organisation. As one EU civil servant commented:

> Of course, again, the tobacco industry are members but some of them have huge membership. But again it's hard to know how influential certain members are and aren't. However, I do know that yeah, the American Chamber of Commerce have taken very pro-tobacco stances.

This is in keeping also with previous studies of the US Chamber of Commerce, which suggest tobacco industry funding and engagement with the Chamber played a major role in its emergence as a political actor in the US and beyond (Katz 2015).

Interviewees also revealed that Bruce Lehman, founder of the International Intellectual Property Institute, wrote to Irish Finance Minister, Michael Noonan TD, and Minister for Jobs, Enterprise and Innovation, Richard Bruton TD, expressing their concerns about the impact of the proposed SP measures on IP rights and highlighting the vital importance of IP for Ireland's knowledge-based economy. Underlying these concerns, there appears to be a suggestion that the Irish government, in enacting measures to protect the health of its people, may incur disinvestment from US-based corporations or deter future investment on which Ireland's economic prosperity depends. As was highlighted above, it should be remembered that this occurred in the midst of Ireland's worst financial crisis in living memory and thus represented a significant deterrent to the government in pursuing their proposed course of action. The decision to target ministries other than the Department of Health can also be seen as an attempt to reframe the issue of SP as a principally economic and commercial issue and to create divisions between different branches of the Irish government. However, these divide-and-rule tactics were resisted by the Irish government in its responses, with the ministries targeted directing correspondence to the Ministry of Health and, in so doing, reinforcing the health framing of the issue.

As well as business interests, interviewees revealed that high-level political actors in the US also wrote to the Irish government and the Irish Ambassador opposing SP. These included US congressmen, senators and governors from tobacco-growing states voicing opposition to Ireland's proposed implementation of SP, on the grounds it would infringe IP laws and facilitate counterfeiting (Beesley 2014b; Carswell 2014). Previous studies of corporate political strategy indicate that politicians with industry facilities or interests in their electoral districts or constituencies, and which depend on this industry activity for jobs and tax revenues, are often targeted by industry actors to represent their interests, and are widely susceptible to their overtures (Hawkins and Holden 2014). This also reflects findings presented in the preceding chapter about industry strategy at the EU level, in which MEPs representing areas with tobacco manufacturing or tobacco-dependent industries were also key lobbying targets. Awareness of this approach is particularly acute in the US, where elected officials are engaged in a constant process of fundraising in order to secure their re-election. In addition to the wider connections between the US and Ireland, this perhaps also explains the willingness of policy actors in the US to lobby overseas governments on issues of interest to the tobacco industry.

The extent of any engagement between those contesting the Irish government's policy and TTCs is unclear. Nonetheless, they consistently articulated positions closely aligned with those of the tobacco industry and strongly opposed to SP. One respondent who followed the debates around SP closely detected at least a high degree of coherence between the messages articulated by the various US actors:

> It looked to me like a well-marshalled, well-organised, quite coherent kind of a campaign, you know? And which seemed to me to be pretty well thought out. There wasn't, it wasn't just by accident, it wasn't just the US Chamber of Commerce, it was the US Chamber of Commerce plus other parties.

The degree of political engagement on the issue of SP also reflected the importance of Ireland in the context of regulatory debates on tobacco packaging in other countries, particularly elsewhere in Europe:

> So I think the precedent-setting dimension was very important because this is a tiny island. The Irish market for cigarettes is small. It's .... a lot of people smoke, it's fine, they make a fine money out of it but this country of four million people, two percent of Europe or whatever, one percent, it's really, really quite small. Why this level, why this intensity of action? Why this very high-level stuff at the level of major business organisations in the US, at the level of, you know, state governors at the level of Capitol Hill at the level of Ambassador? Why is that? Really, the only explanation is the precedent-setting dimension.

Finally, the clear focus of engagement from the US-based actors was on the issue of IP, a core TTC argument against SP, but one which potentially could, at least theoretically, affect actors from other sectors. This facilitated the involvement of business organisations in lobbying against these specifically tobacco-related measures under the auspices of a wider concern about the undermining of IP rights in general. It also facilitated the engagement of Irish umbrella business organisations, such as the Irish Business and Employers Confederation (IBEC), in the debates on SP in ways amenable to TTC interests. Similarly, it facilitated the engagement of political actors in correspondence with the Irish government on a point of law and regulatory 'good practice'.

Local Knowledge, Global Significance

As argued above and in our previous work (Hawkins et al. 2018), the industry has an over-arching global strategy to block the introduction of increased labelling requirements and packaging restrictions. However, this strategy is implemented in subtly different ways tailored to the specificities of the local political, cultural and institutional context. Whilst many of the arguments used may be similar, and many of the lobbying tactics employed, such as the use of political consultancies and PR companies, may be identical in different political settings, their arguments will be articulated with local 'accents' and the specific vehicles identified for the industry message will vary depending on local conditions, in order to maximise their effectiveness. For example, it is a key component of tobacco industry strategy to seek meetings with key political actors at the highest possible level, despite the political sensitivities around this and the obligations beholden on policy-makers under Article 5.3 of the FCTC. In Ireland, the industry was able to secure a meeting with Taoiseach Enda Kenny and three senior ministers by utilising long-standing connections between a specific Dublin-based PR consultancy and the ruling Fine Gael party, and the personal relationship between the head of this organisation and the Taoiseach himself (Cullen 2013).

Before his death in 2015 Bill O'Herlihy was both a much-loved sports commentator on Irish television and the head of O'Herlihy Communications which, according to interview respondents, had previously worked on behalf of the tobacco industry, and which had acted for Fine Gael on a *pro bono* basis during the preceding Irish general election. Through his engagement with Fine Gael politics O'Herlihy had also had a long-standing personal relationship with Kenny. O'Herlihy facilitated a meeting between the Taoiseach, the Minister of Finance, Michael Noonan, and the Minister for Justice and Equality, Alan Shatter, and the Irish Tobacco Manufacturers Association (ITMAC) and various tobacco company chief executives in May 2013, ostensibly to discuss the problem of illicit trade (McGreevy 2013, 2014). The possibility of a meeting between the tobacco industry and senior ministers in a country with such an impressive record on tobacco control was explained by interviewees as being a direct result of the personal relationship between Kenny and O'Herlihy. Health Minister James Reilly, who was leading on the SP legislation, was apparently not invited, but indicated that he would have refused to attend in any case. This is perhaps just the clearest example of the TTCs' use of political consultancies and connections with Fine Gael, including former party staffers now employed by TTCs, which respondents reported. It is arguable, however, that the meeting represented a strategic miscalculation by the tobacco industry (Beesley 2013b) given the controversy to which it gave rise. The government announced its plans to proceed with SP soon afterwards.

Tobacco industry actors thus demonstrated a highly nuanced understanding of the political terrain of Irish politics and the relationships between key individuals in seeking and gaining access to key decision-makers. However, the significance of the meeting extends far beyond their attempts to influence Irish policy debates. A meeting with a head of government in a state widely regarded as hostile to the industry provided the industry with significant political capital in its campaigns against SP and labelling requirements elsewhere. The documentation of such a meeting could be used to lobby governments elsewhere for similar meetings and to undermine attempts to marginalise TTC actors from policy debates under the auspices of FCTC Article 5.3. As one NGO representative commented:

> The tobacco industry are very, very clear, you know, if this is a global thing and particularly if this is, you know, if you think about the fact that [...], Ireland is definitely seen as a leader in tobacco control. So the fact that the tobacco industry is in a position to meet with the prime minister of such a tobacco-control-leading country is going to be a feather in the cap for them. And they yeah absolutely they will go to other countries and say – and in fact I've noted that that was probably used in like that … it was actually used in letters as well from the tobacco industry or from friends of the tobacco industry to the government around the time of plain packaging as well. You know, kind of "as you would've heard around the time of your meeting with the tobacco industry, you would have heard about smuggling" or something like that. So yeah they would absolutely know that this was a feather in the cap for them.

Whilst the meeting with Kenny may have provided important political capital for the industry for use in policy debates elsewhere in Ireland and beyond, the political controversy surrounding the meeting, following its revelation in the media, redoubled the political pressure on the government to proceed with SP both from health advocacy organisations and key actors inside the government committed to the policy, including Health Minister James Reilly.

Third-Party Lobbying

Alongside IP arguments the other principle argument against SP was that it would facilitate the illicit trade in cigarettes. Whilst the arguments on IP were made by business and law associations, both domestic and overseas, arguments against illicit trade were made by retailers and their relevant trade associations. These were allied to concerns about the negative economic impact of SP on their businesses. Newsagents and corner shop owners were a potentially effective conduit for this argument. As small businesses at the heart of local communities, they represented the very antithesis of the global corporations of the tobacco industry, whose interests were actually most directly affected by the proposed laws. However, respondents were widely of the opinion that retailers were being targeted by the tobacco industry and supplied with materials and messages about the adverse effects of SP. In particular, they were used to raise concerns about the lost revenues for convenience store owners as a result of illicit and counterfeit products, which TTCs argued would increase in volume following the introduction of SP. When asked about the arguments employed by the industry against SP, a representative from a Dublin-based NGO commented:

> It's the same ones they've made everywhere else. And they always are the same arguments. But the usual ones like the one about smuggling particularly. That's what they went really heavy on. That's what the media tends to be interested in so they used that in kind of the media circles. But they also used it in, with retailers. That was certainly their focus with retailers. And like we know that one of the companies was doing round-table meetings across the country with retailers. Apparently Ireland's quite unusual in that we have a tobacco rep system where there's an awful lot of reps for the number of retailers in parts of the country. So the reps are going in and visiting retailers on a very regular basis. And we did hear from certain retailers that they were being given leaflets and information basically relating plain packaging to smuggling and how it was going to damage their business. So you know,

> even asking them if they would contact their local politician and talk to them about why it could be really damaging to them.

The use of retailers as a conduit for this illicit-trade argument was corroborated by multiple respondents. This was perhaps most obvious in the creation of the 'astroturf' organisation Retailers Against Smuggling, funded by the Irish Tobacco Manufacturers' Advisory Committee and other corporate sponsors, which became a focal point for industry-sponsored activities against SP. According to the respondent, their position contrasted with that of Retail Ireland, which took a more measured stance on SP and, despite raising some concerns about the potential impact of the policy on their members, were conscious not to be seen to be opposing public health measures. Larger retailers, such as the main supermarket chains, were largely absent from the debate as individual actors, however. In addition to domestic organisations, there were also interventions in the debate by UK-based organisations:

> We also noticed that Ireland suddenly became very interesting to a lot of organisations who hadn't been that bothered by Ireland. [...] And suddenly they became very active in media here.

Retail organisations in Ireland that were opposed to SP targeted members of the Irish parliament (TDs) in an attempt to influence their positions on the law. A representative of another public health NGO explained the role they had to play in assisting TDs targeted by local retailers:

> So we would've made sure that we were in and around Leinster House meeting who we've considered to be key backbenchers. So this [TD] and she told us that she met all the retailers in her constituency. Now, she said she was holding the line on plain packaging, there was absolutely no question about it, but she asked us for like what's the counter argument. What's the argument really for plain packaging? And we were able to, obviously, give her the correct information on illicit, on the level of illicit and that kind of thing. [...]. But really what they were saying was this is going to kill off our sector. Now, it's not going to happen. Do you know what I mean? It's just the usual. Of course, we point out they use this argument in Australia, it's the same argument everywhere.

This was reflected by other NGOs who highlighted the targeting of rural TDs, in whose communities small retailers may play a particularly important role.

Domestic Law Firms

Similar arguments to those made by actors from other countries about the infringement of IP rights were made in the domestic sphere. Here also, these were made not only by the tobacco industry and their trade associations, but by professional bodies with apparently no direct association with the tobacco industry, but with a broader concern about the unintended consequences of the SP measures. This was perhaps most obviously the case with the Law Society of Ireland's Intellectual Property Committee during the Joint Oireachtas Committee Hearings into the proposed SP legislation in January 2014. Several respondents raised concerns about the links between the IP Committee and the tobacco industry. Moreover, whilst the Law Society has a long and well-documented history, the IP Committee was of more recent standing. As one NGO respondent notes:

> And then around that time we discovered that the Law Society of Ireland had a sub-committee on intellectual property. Never been heard of before, so we looked it up anyway and we discovered that it had only been in existence for less than a year, and that it was being chaired by people who'd worked for the tobacco industry.

The arguments presented by the Law Society to the Oireachtas Committee closely mirrored those made by the tobacco industry in Ireland and elsewhere. Moreover, their intervention seemed to move beyond the narrow remit of IP into other areas of direct concern to TTCs, but less obviously within the IP Committee's expertise, such as the impact of SP on illicit trade. As one NGO respondent commented:

> The first thing that we noticed was around the time of the public submissions around plain packaging the Law Society had put in a submission on plain packaging. Now when we took a look initially at what they had said, the first thing that we noticed is that it didn't come from the Law Society itself but it came from a Committee on Intellectual Property. [...] and when you read the actual submission by the Intellectual Property Committee of the Law Society of Ireland [...] they go into how plain packaging is going to affect

> smuggling rates. Now I don't know about you but to me lawyers are not experts in smuggling.

An Irish politician who observed the Oireachtas Committee hearings noted close similarities between the arguments presented by the Law Society and tobacco industry positions:

> I think for me I suppose the real thing that got me was we have the Law Society of Ireland. And it came in under the Law Society of Ireland. And when reading their submission a few sentences jumped out that I went, whoa! That's tobacco industry sentences!

The same respondent also confirmed that there were connections between key personnel on the IP Committee and tobacco industry actors:

> So I started then to look at who was on this committee. And other members of the committee, you know, you had people who did the trademarks for the tobacco company, you had somebody who had only up until recently worked for a tobacco company for quite a period was now a solicitor and was there.

As described in the previous chapter, it appears that law firms with tobacco industry clients may serve as a potential conduit for industry objectives on key tobacco policy debates, in ways which are not obviously associated with the industry itself.

Tobacco companies retained the services of a range of law firms and barristers to represent their interests during the passage of the SP legislation. According to interview respondents, the effect of this was not only to ensure that TTCs had significant resources to dedicate to scrutinising and potentially challenging the legislation, but to reduce the pool of available legal and other professional services firms available to public health actors and the government to represent their own interests.

Legal Challenges

As the legislation to enact SP moved through the legislative process, tobacco industry actors, in highlighting the alleged infringement of IP rights, made it clear to the Irish government that they would mount legal challenges to the proposed laws. This included legal opinions prepared by counsel for TTCs such as Philip Morris sent to the Irish government outlining the potentially deleterious costs of a successful legal challenge to SP.

In keeping with the industry narratives about the expropriation of their IP, explicit parallels were drawn between the Irish case and the on-going legal processes against Australia. This caused internal discussion within the Irish government about whether the legislation should proceed whilst the legal cases against Australia were still on-going. As one respondent with knowledge of the policy process commented, there were significant concerns in Ireland about the potential implications of introducing SP in Ireland and the possibility of similar legal challenges to their measures:

> There was concern about the legal challenge and that concern was highlighted over and over again. We were actually in a weaker position then than we are now because we didn't have real world data out of Australia like now. [... two government officials] went out there and said, "sure, they took on the Australian government and lost, do we have anything to worry about here?" But we do. The copyrights in the Irish Constitution are a lot stronger than the framework in Australia. The other thing, there was also a bit of a chill factor in terms of the World Trade Organization [...] "will we wait until this... until Australia to see how they get on in the World Trade Organization?" [...] So that was, you know, that kind of stuff just falls into your head immediately and we know it's part of ... we now know it's part of the industry tactics.

Ultimately, however, the threat of litigation, both domestically and under international trade laws, was unable to stymie the progress of the Irish legislation on SP. At this stage, the legal arguments of the tobacco industry switched to more concrete actions against the Irish government. Initially, this took the form of a letter to the Irish government threatening legal action. As the previous respondent continued:

> We had gone through the Seanad [Upper House of Parliament], we had gone through the second stage in the Daíl [the Lower House]. We had notified in Europe [...]. And it was just about to come to an end and [the government] got a remarkable legal letter from JTI [Japan Tobacco International] where they decided to throw the kitchen sink at us and tell us they want it in writing within ten days, that we're not going to progress this legislation any further in our parliament, or they'll take legal action around this sort of stuff. So not only were they telling us that we couldn't pass the legislation, they were trying to dictate to us the pace the legislation could pass through our parliament and which part of the legislation process we could bring it to... so it was a totally outlandish letter.

However, this approach proved to be a strategic miscalculation by the industry. Not only did it fail to deter the government from progressing with their proposals, it arguably strengthened the resolve of policy-makers not to be intimidated by what they perceived to be industry threats. Furthermore, the public support for the policy also appeared to be buttressed by the industry's actions. The previous respondent commented:

> This caused huge PR damage to the tobacco industry because it really turned the journalists against them and I think it really turned the public against them. I saw four polls on plain packaging in Ireland. The first one was a Eurobarometer one and I think it showed support [for SP] of seventy something percent, early seventies. Then there was two Irish Cancer Society ones. […] And the support in the Cancer Society polls showed it falling. I think the first one maybe sixty-seven percent and the second one was sixty-two percent. So they were having an impact on public support […] But then after all the litigation they commissioned another Eurobarometer poll and it showed support at eighty-four percent […] So the public didn't like their tactics at all, they were shot on them.

A further respondent in the public health sector also suggested that the highly combative approach taken by the tobacco industry may reflect the lack of local knowledge, or cultural sensitivity, on the part of the particular company leading the action. It was suggested that JTI executives may have lacked an appreciation of how the tone of their approach would play out in the Irish context and that other companies, with longer standing connections to the Irish market, may have realised the potential hazards of taking this approach and devised different strategies.

Following the enactment of SP legislation by the Irish government in March 2015, JTI Ireland launched a legal challenge in the Irish Commercial Court to prevent the introduction of the measures. JTI claimed that SP could undermine the functioning of the European single market by creating differential packaging requirements and imposing a barrier on trade between member states (O'Faolain 2015). As an EU member state, they argued, Ireland could not unilaterally introduce SP, which went beyond what was required to successfully transpose the EU TPD into domestic law. Moreover, the measures would go against the stated harmonisation objectives of the TPD. The Irish government sought to have this referred to the Court of Justice of the European Union (CJEU) for preliminary ruling on relevant points of EU law. This motion was declined by the Commercial Court, however, on the basis that similar action had been taken against

SP measures by Philip Morris International (PMI) and British American Tobacco (BAT) in the UK High Court and that this case had already been referred to the CJEU (*The Irish Times* 2015). Consequently, the legality of the policy in the EU context would be established by the outcome of that case, with the Irish courts adhering also to the ruling in that case (Cullen 2015). A press release by JTI summarised their position:

> We welcome the court's decision today. From the outset, we said that it was unnecessary to refer these questions because the CJEU is already looking at a similar referral from the UK Courts. The outcome of this UK case will be absolutely critical to the right of any EU Member State to introduce plain packaging, which is why we asked the Government to wait for a decision before enacting the legislation. An Irish referral would also have had the potential to delay the European Court's decision, which is something we want to avoid. Strict new EU tobacco regulations are scheduled to come into force across all Member States in May 2016, so we are keen to see this issue resolved as quickly as possible. (Shelf Life 2015)

The rationale for opposing a separate Irish referral to the CJEU is a point of some conjecture. It was suggested by respondents and in media coverage that the second referral to the CJEU may have complicated and delayed the process in both contexts. JTI seemed keen to have the case in Ireland heard, and resolved in their favour, prior to the planned commencement of the policy in May 2016, in the hope of preventing standardised packs from hitting the shelves. The arrival of SP would have had an important psychological effect on the policy debate and rendered the debate tangible to decision-makers and the wider public. Given biases towards the status quo, repealing rather than preventing its introduction would have been a greater challenge for the industry.

However, one actor intimately involved in the policy process suggested that this may have been an example of 'venue shifting' by TTCs to a decision-making setting where their objectives were more likely to be achieved. Tobacco companies may have felt more able to influence the process through the UK courts than via the Irish courts because of the high public and political support for SP in Ireland. Multiple respondents also reiterated the overwhelming degree of consensus which exists in Ireland, amongst both the political class and the wider population, in favour of tobacco-control measures. As one respondent commented:

> It is non-political. No, there isn't a... I would say over the years, the NGO community have absolutely won tobacco, hands down, in persuading every elected representative that tobacco and tobacco industries are bad.

Ireland had been the first country in Europe to introduce legislation for smoke-free public spaces and the Minister responsible for that, Micheál Martin, was at the time of the SP legislation the leader of the main opposition Fianna Fáil party. The UK by contrast had shown significant reluctance to lead in Europe on both smoke-free legislation and SP, with devolved administrations in Scotland committing politically to both policies in advance of Westminster. In the summer of 2013, the UK government announced that the introduction of SP would be delayed—a decision ultimately reversed following an outcry by health actors. Speculation subsequently circulated suggesting that David Cameron's election strategist, Lynton Crosby—who also runs a consultancy that has worked on behalf of Philip Morris International—may have influenced the decision to delay SP, a claim Crosby has denied (Wintour 2013).

The CJEU ruled on 4 May 2016 that SP was in keeping with EU single-market law and permissible within the remit of the TPD, paving the way for the introduction of SP in both Ireland and throughout the EU. On 19 May 2016 the application by TTCs for a judicial review of the UK government's SP laws was rejected by the High Court in London (Ross 2016). Subsequent appeals by BAT and JTI were also rejected by the UK Court of Appeal and the Supreme Court. However, the legal remedies available to TTCs to challenge SP legislation in Ireland may not have been exhausted. Given that the focus of the legal challenge in Ireland was to do explicitly with the legality of the TPD and the compatibility of SP with the objectives of the Directive, the possibility remained open for a further challenge to the Irish government on the grounds of IP rights under the Irish constitution, although such a challenge did not ultimately materialise, perhaps because a challenge to the Australian government under its consitution had previously been unsuccessful. The use of legal challenges in Ireland is in keeping with established industry strategy to delay the introduction of packaging restrictions where it is not possible to block them fully (Hawkins and Holden 2016; Holden and Hawkins 2017; Hawkins et al. 2018; Jarman 2015). A further effect of legal challenges is the demand it places on government resources and therefore the effect it has not only on potentially delaying the policy under challenge but the wider development of tobacco-control measures. One respondent highlighted the inertia of current policy debates and how the strategy on SP mirrored the approach taken by the industry previously to challenge smoke-free legislation:

> I suspect, I don't know this, I suspect the reasons that the regulations aren't ready for the [ban on smoking in] cars is that these people are tied up doing this bloody thing. That suits the industry and it also suits them to prolong it. The last big thing we had was of the law on the smoke free and some aspect of it. And they kept it going to three years. At the end of the day they put their hands up and said no it's OK we'll drop it. They had tied up everyone including all the advocates.

In contrast to the Australian case, respondents reported that, whilst references were made to WTO law in the context of arguments about IP put forward to oppose the policy, there appeared to be little indication from the industry that there would arise claims against Ireland within the WTO, or that the industry would seek to initiate action under investor-state dispute settlement (ISDS) mechanisms in bilateral investment treaties (BITs). This again underlines the propensity of TTCs to tailor their political strategies to oppose packaging regulations to the specific political context in which they are operating. Ireland's membership of the EU provided a degree of cover from WTO challenges, as it would be the EU, as opposed to Ireland individually, against whom procedures must be taken. Whilst WTO member states were prepared to initiate WTO disputes against Australia's SP laws, facilitated at least in part by the financial support of the tobacco industry (Eckhardt et al. 2016), there would be significant disincentives for states to take such measures against the world's largest trading bloc unless it were firmly in the country's core economic interests to do so. Moreover, bringing such a challenge directly against Ireland and the EU may have been seen as superfluous by the industry, with the Australian case still under consideration by the WTO. An industry-favourable ruling in the Australian case would have created a precedent in WTO law which could then have subsequently been used as the basis of a dispute with Ireland, and other EU member states considering the introduction of SP. As such, there was no need for TTCs to expend financial and political capital at this stage to lobby WTO member states to challenge the EU directly on SP, when Australia could be pursued as a test case. Moreover, as the Australian case continued it could be used to lobby governments to delay introducing SP until its resolution, and may have already deterred other states from initiating similar legislation. The EU context also meant there was another body of law under which national policies could be challenged, which was not available to the industry in Australia. It appears then that the TTCs took a strategic decision to utilise the mechanisms of legal recourse available to them that were most likely to succeed in each instance, in a sophisticated process of venue shopping.

Summary

The Irish government, and Health Minister James Riley in particular, demonstrated strong political commitment to tobacco control at the domestic and European levels. Riley played a vital role in the passage of the EU TPD during the Irish Presidency of the Council and led efforts to introduce SP in Ireland. These efforts at the national level were assisted by the recognition of member states' right to move beyond the packaging requirements laid down in the TPD. Thus, the domestic policy debates in Ireland cannot be separated from Ireland's role at the European level in helping to secure legal recognition of the possibility of SP at member-state level. More generally, developments in Ireland need to be understood in the context of Ireland's position within a system of multi-level governance within the EU. Despite provisions in the TPD, and the compatibility of the Irish SP policy with EU single-market law, the industry used EU legal processes to try to block or delay the implementation of SP in Ireland and the UK. Alongside the use of legal challenges, which mirror tactics employed in Australia and Uruguay, TTCs tailored their political strategy to the specific Irish context. They used EU-level actors and the close economic and political ties with the US in an attempt to prevent and delay the policy. As such, the Irish experience of introducing SP confirms that, while TTCs have highly coordinated global political strategies, these are adapted to national settings, reflecting the principle 'think global, act local' (Hawkins et al. 2018).

Bibliography

Beesley, A. (2013a, May 24). Taoiseach heavily criticised for meeting tobacco lobby. *The Irish Times*. Available at https://www.irishtimes.com/news/politics/taoiseach-heavily-criticised-for-meeting-tobacco-lobby-1.1404690. Accessed 1 March 2019.

Beesley, A. (2013b, May 23). Taoiseach holds formal talks with tobacco industry. *The Irish Times*. Available at https://www.irishtimes.com/news/taoiseach-holds-formal-talks-with-tobacco-industry-1.1403487?mode=sample&auth-failed=1&pw-origin=https%3A%2F%2Fwww.irishtimes.com%2Fnews%2Ftaoiseach-holds-formal-talks-with-tobacco-industry-1.1403487. Accessed 1 March 2019.

Beesley, A. (2014a, June 10). Reilly to seek Cabinet approval for plain tobacco packaging. *The Irish Times*. Available at https://www.irishtimes.com/news/politics/reilly-to-seek-cabinet-approval-for-plain-tobacco-packaging-1.1826443. Accessed 1 March 2019.

Beesley, A. (2014b, April 5). US business lobbies urge Kenny to rethink tobacco packaging. *The Irish Times*. Available at https://www.irishtimes.com/news/politics/us-business-lobbies-urge-kenny-to-rethink-tobacco-packaging-1.1751038. Accessed 1 March 2019.

Beesley, A. (2014c, June 18). Tobacco lobby steps up campaign against plain packaging. *The Irish Times*. Available at https://www.irishtimes.com/news/politics/tobacco-lobby-steps-up-campaign-against-plain-packaging-1.1835924. Accessed 1 March 2019.

Carswell, S. (2014, September 25). US governor urges Government not to use plain tobacco packaging. *The Irish Times*. Available at https://www.irishtimes.com/news/politics/us-governor-urges-government-not-to-use-plain-tobacco-packaging-1.1941863. Accessed 1 March 2019.

Cullen, P. (2013, September 9). Five former Fine Gael aides working for tobacco industry. *The Irish Times*. Available at https://www.irishtimes.com/news/ireland/irish-news/five-former-fine-gael-aides-working-for-tobacco-industry-1.1520426?mode = sample&auth-failed = 1&pw-origin = https%3A%2F%2Fwww.irishtimes.com%2Fnews%2Fireland%2Firish-news%2Ffive-former-fine-gael-aides-working-for-tobacco-industry-1.1520426. Accessed 1 March 2019.

Cullen, P. (2015, December 23). European Court of Justice rules in favour of plain packaging directive for cigarettes. *The Irish Times*. Available at https://www.irishtimes.com/news/health/european-court-of-justice-rules-in-favour-of-plain-packaging-directive-for-cigarettes-1.2475981?mode = sample&auth-failed = 1&pw-origin = https%3A%2F%2Fwww.irishtimes.com%2Fnews%2Fhealth%2Feuropean-court-of-justice-rules-in-favour-of-plain-packaging-directive-for-cigarettes-1.2475981. Accessed 1 March 2019.

Eckhardt, J., Holden, C., & Callard, C. (2016). Tobacco Control and the World Trade Organization: Mapping Member States' Positions after the Framework Convention on Tobacco Control. *Tobacco Control, 25*, 692–698.

European Commission. (2014). *Notification Detail: Public Health (Standardised Packaging of Tobacco) Bill 2014*. European Commission. Available at http://ec.europa.eu/growth/tools-databases/tris/en/search/?trisaction=search.detail&year=2014&num=277. Accessed 1 March 2019.

Hammond, D. (2014). *Standardized packaging of tobacco products evidence review prepared on behalf of the Irish Department of Health*. Available at http://health.gov.ie/wp-content/uploads/2014/06/2014-Ireland-Plain-Pack-Main-Report-Final-Report-July-26.pdf. Accessed 2 March 2018.

Hawkins, B., & Holden, C. (2014). "Water dripping on stone"? Industry lobbying and UK alcohol policy. *Policy & Politics, 42*(1), 55–70.

Hawkins, B., & Holden, C. (2016). A corporate veto on health policy? Global constitutionalism and investor-state dispute settlement. *Journal of Health Politics, Policy and Law, 13,* 1–19.

Hawkins, B., Holden, C., & Mackinder, S. (2018). A multi-level, multi-jurisdictional strategy: Transnational tobacco companies' attempts to obstruct tobacco packaging restrictions. *Global Public Health.* https://doi.org/10.1080/17441692.2018.1446997.

Holden, C., & Hawkins, B. (2017). Law, market building and public health in the European Union. *Global Social Policy,* 1–17.

Jarman, H. (2015). *The politics of trade and tobacco control.* Basingstoke: Palgrave Macmillan.

Katz, A. (2015). *The influence machine: The US chamber of commerce and the corporate capture of American life.* New York: Speigel & Grau.

McEnroe, J. (2014a, August 12). Plain tobacco packets 'will hurt recovery'. *Irish Examiner.* Available at https://www.irishexaminer.com/ireland/plain-tobacco-packets-will-hurt-recovery-279302.html. Accessed 1 March 2019.

McEnroe, J. (2014b, August 12). Plain Cigarette Packaging: A burning issue in the EU. *Irish Examiner.* Available at https://www.irishexaminer.com/viewpoints/analysis/plain-cigarette-packaging-a-burning-issue-in-the-eu-279196.html. Accessed 1 March 2019.

McGreevy, R. (2013, September 9). O'Herlihy thanks Deenihan for 'terrific' help in getting access to Ministers. *The Irish Times.* Available at https://www.irishtimes.com/news/ireland/irish-news/o-herlihy-thanked-deenihan-for-terrific-help-in-getting-access-to-ministers-1.1520428?mode = sample&auth-failed = 1&pw-origin = https%3A%2F%2Fwww.irishtimes.com%2Fnews%2Fireland%2Firish-news%2Fo-herlihy-thanked-deenihan-for-terrific-help-in-getting-access-to-ministers-1.1520428. Accessed 1 March 2019.

McGreevy, R. (2014, June 11). Bill O'Herlihy defends role as lobbyist for tobacco industry. *The Irish Times.* Available at https://www.irishtimes.com/news/ireland/irish-news/bill-o-herlihy-defends-role-as-lobbyist-for-tobacco-industry-1.1828430?mode = sample&auth-failed = 1&pw-origin = https%3A%2F%2Fwww.irishtimes.com%2Fnews%2Fireland%2Firish-news%2Fbill-o-herlihy-defends-role-as-lobbyist-for-tobacco-industry-1.1828430. Accessed 1 March 2019.

O'Connor, N. (2015). Minister Reilly rejects criticism of his tobacco plans. *The Independent.* Available at https://www.independent.ie/irish-news/politics/minister-reilly-rejects-criticism-of-his-tobacco-plans-30966056.html. Accessed 1 March 2019.

O'Faolain, A. (2015). State wants tobacco packaging challenge referred to EU court. *The Irish Times.* Available at https://www.irishtimes.com/business/manufacturing/state-wants-tobacco-packaging-challenge-referred-to-eu-court-1.2190636?mode = sample&auth-failed = 1&pw-origin = https%3A%

2F%2Fwww.irishtimes.com%2Fbusiness%2Fmanufacturing%2Fstate-wants-tobacco-packaging-challenge-referred-to-eu-court-1.2190636. Accessed 1 March 2019.

Ross, A. (2016, May 19). British American Tobacco plan to appeal plain packaging rule. *The Daily Echo*. Available at https://www.dailyecho.co.uk/news/14504332.Southampton_tobacco_firm_plan_to_appeal_plain_packaging_rule/. Accessed 1 March 2019.

Shelf Life. (2015, July 7). *JTI Ireland welcomes Commercial Court ruling in plain packaging case*. Shelf Life. Available at https://www.shelflife.ie/jti-ireland-welcomes-commercial-court-ruling-in-plain-packaging-case/. Accessed 1 March 2019.

The Irish Times. (2015, July 8). State loses bid to have tobacco questions referred to EU court. *Irish Times*. Available at https://www.irishtimes.com/business/health-pharma/state-loses-bid-to-have-tobacco-questions-referred-to-eu-court-1.2276765?mode = sample&auth-failed = 1&pw-origin = https%3A%2F%2Fwww.irishtimes.com%2Fbusiness%2Fhealth-pharma%2Fstate-loses-bid-to-have-tobacco-questions-referred-to-eu-court-1.2276765. Accessed 1 March 2019.

Wintour, P. (2013, July 23). Lynton Crosby: I have never discussed tobacco issues with Cameron. *The Guardian*. Available at https://www.theguardian.com/politics/2013/jul/23/lynton-crosby-tobacco-issues-david-cameron. Accessed 22 October 2019.

CHAPTER 5

Policy Transfer and Transnational NGO Networks

Abstract This chapter focuses on the roles of non-governmental organisations (NGOs) in the adoption of standardised packaging (SP) for cigarettes in Ireland and the adoption of the revised Tobacco Products Directive (TPD) by the European Union (EU). Transnational networks between NGOs and other policy actors in Australia, Ireland, the United Kingdom (UK) and at the EU level are identified as facilitating three types of policy learning between jurisdictions: horizontal-consecutive policy learning, characterising the relationship between Australian and Irish NGOs; horizontal-concurrent policy learning, characterising the relationship between Irish and UK NGOs; and vertical policy learning, characterising the relationship between NGOs active at the EU level and those based in member states such as Ireland. The latter two types of policy learning may be bi-directional.

Keywords Standardised tobacco packaging · Plain packaging · Non-governmental organisations · European Union · Policy learning · Policy transfer

The story of standardised packaging (SP) in Europe, like that of tobacco control more generally, cannot be told without significant reference to the role of public health and tobacco-control actors in civil society in bringing such measures onto the policy agenda and supporting governments'

B. Hawkins et al., *The Battle for Standardised Cigarette Packaging in Europe*, Palgrave Studies in Public Health Policy Research,
https://doi.org/10.1007/978-3-030-31034-9_5

attempts to enact them in law. Agenda setting is a key dimension of the policy process and the role of non-governmental organisations (NGOs) working on tobacco-related issues in identifying SP as an effective tobacco-control policy around which the sector could unite, and bringing it to the attention of key policy-makers, was vital in securing its introduction in Ireland, the United Kingdom (UK) and, subsequently, other European Union (EU) member states. In the face of significant opposition by the tobacco industry, these actors played a vital role in highlighting the scale of tobacco-related harms, and the efficacy of SP as a means of reducing these and preventing smoking initiation, especially amongst young people. Their advocacy work focused on explaining the merits of the policy to both policy-makers and the wider public, whose support for the policy would be vital in securing its successful adoption. Furthermore, the on-going commitment of the NGO sector was essential in supporting the passage of SP-related legislation and its successful implementation in the face of determined efforts by the tobacco industry to prevent and delay this.

In this chapter, we examine the role played by public health and civil society actors in securing the introduction of SP in Ireland, and the role played by similar organisations in other settings to support this process via transnational NGO networks. This chapter follows the organisational logic of the book more widely in seeing Ireland as the political 'leader' on SP in Europe, showing the firmest commitment to the introduction of the policy. The focus on Ireland reflects not just the fact that it was the first EU member state to propose and enact SP, but that it was the country that offered the greatest political leadership on the issue. Given the vital role that the Irish government played in the adoption of the EU Tobacco Products Directive (TPD) during its Presidency of the Council—and in previous tobacco-control debates such as the introduction of smoke-free public spaces—Irish policy-makers and civil society actors sought to embed their reputation as public health innovators by leading the way on SP in Europe.

Following developments in Ireland, the UK announced similar intentions to adopt SP. The size of the UK market and the political weight of the UK as a global health actor means that this, not least from an industry perspective, could be considered a more significant development. Moreover, UK NGOs also played a vital role in advocating and supporting the policy and deserve much credit for its eventual adoption in the UK. Yet the UK government may not have adopted SP without the pressure to do so which resulted from Ireland's commitment to the policy. Equivocations on SP by David Cameron's coalition government, even after its announcement of the policy, speak to the very different levels of governmental commitment to the issue on either side of the Irish Sea. The Irish government's commitment to pressing ahead with the policy is therefore highly significant. As will be examined below, both public health actors and the tobacco industry, which opposed SP's introduction, believed this would lead to the 'domino effect' we have subsequently seen, with other member states following suit. Holding the line on SP across the EU and, if possible, demonstrating its consistency or otherwise with EU law, was thus of vital importance for actors on both sides of the debate. For these reasons, we focus our analysis around processes in Ireland, and the efforts of Irish civil-society actors to implement SP, but highlight also the crucial role played by civil-society actors in Australia and the UK in supporting their activities.

We draw on theories of policy transfer and multi-level governance set out in Chapter 2 to explain how these global and European NGO and policy networks were a key factor in overcoming policy-makers' reticence to pursue SP in the context of vehement industry opposition, and thus in securing the introduction of the policy in Ireland and the UK. We examine the ways in which government and civil society actors in Australia shared their experiences of the previous legislative battle over SP there with colleagues in Ireland and played a vital role in shaping their successful advocacy strategy. We identify also the significance of concurrent political developments on SP in the UK, knowledge sharing between NGOs, and the support offered by the greater resources available to tobacco-control advocates in the much larger neighbouring polity. Finally, we place events in Ireland in the context of wider European policy networks.

Civil Society and Public Health Coordination in Ireland

As in Australia, civil society actors played a key role in the development of SP in Ireland. Their role was to provide evidence and information about the policy, designed to inform key policy-makers attempting to push the legislation on SP through Parliament, and to convince the wider public of its merits. Their strategy involved framing the debate as a health issue and a children's rights issue, drawing on the experiences of related policy debates in other settings. At the heart of this campaign were a series of inter-relationships between NGOs and other policy actors. There was coordination and cooperation between the domestic NGOs working on smoking issues; between NGOs in the tobacco-control sector and those working in other areas, such as children's charities; between domestic NGOs and the Ministry of Health; between public health actors and NGOs in Australia and Ireland and between those in the UK and Ireland. We categorise the relationship between Australian and Irish NGOs as an example of *horizontal-consecutive policy learning*; the interactions between UK and Irish NGOs meanwhile are an example of *horizontal-concurrent policy learning*. This takes place in the context of a system of multi-level governance within the EU, which facilitates *vertical policy learning* between policy actors at different levels of governance. These processes of policy learning occur via horizontally and vertically integrated NGO networks. In this section we examine the inter-relationship between domestic NGOs and other policy actors in Ireland before moving on to examine the horizontal and vertical engagement with external actors in the sections which follow.

Domestic NGO Networks

A key aspect of the campaign to introduce SP in Ireland was the cooperation and coordination of the main domestic public health NGOs working on issues related to smoking and tobacco control. Principal among these were the Irish Heart Foundation (IHF) and the Irish Cancer Society (ICS), as well as Action on Smoking and Heath (ASH) Ireland. As a respondent from the IHF commented, the main tobacco-control NGOs work closely in tandem with one another in order to maximise the impact of their work given the limited resources available to them:

> Well, I suppose, like ourselves, the Cancer Society [...], and there's ASH as well. But we'd be the two kind of leading organisations that do the kind of advocacy work around tobacco control in Ireland. And like in the Heart Foundation, there's basically like one other person working on this area [...].
>
> [...] ourselves and the Cancer Society working in tandem, because that's what we find on tobacco is the most, has been the most successful for us. And we do the same things, right? You know, budget issues and all that. We tend to run tobacco and all that together.

On the issue of SP the cooperation between the NGOs became perhaps more structured than on other issues. As the respondent continues:

> So the strategy I suppose was that ourselves and the Cancer Society would establish this coalition and it was kind of a loose coalition, we're calling it 'The Standardised Packaging Coalition', it never had any kind of official name or anything. And we had pretty regular meetings over the kind of year-and-a-half period of the plain packaging with that group and it was about, it was providing quite a lot of information so that then those organisations […] were comfortable about the issue.

Presenting a united front in terms of policy messaging and creating a single point of contact for policy-makers was an effective way of achieving access to key decision-makers. As the previous respondent elaborated:

> So literally, like having regular meetings and actually being coordinated, coming out with joint documents, which is fine. It's just a lot stronger. And the political system likes it as well. They like to know that there's one kind of core position that's held and we would be seen as the main tobacco-control organisation so that if, you know, from the NGO sector, so if we were saying it and if we're both saying the same thing, they feel comfortable.

While the unity of messaging and the coordinated approach within what were seen as the main tobacco-control NGOs was of vital importance, anti-smoking campaigners recognised the importance of involving voices from outside their narrow policy domain in the debate. This meant generalising the importance of SP to other areas and securing supporting voices beyond the tobacco-control community to engage bodies such as the Irish Thoracic Society, and the Asthma Society. Perhaps of greatest significance in this case, the engagement of children's charities was vital in framing SP as a children's rights issue. As the previous respondent commented:

> As I said, you don't want the same voices all of the time. So people in the coalition were very useful and very helpful in doing an awful lot of media work and, as I said, focusing on that child aspect […]. I mean, we learned certainly from the children's organisations as well because they kind of take a more children's rights approach to policy issues. It's not something that really happens in Ireland in terms of a kind of a kind of rights-based approach and health policy.

As the respondent makes clear, engagement with children's charities led tobacco-control NGOs to develop their policy-influencing strategies and evolve their understanding of their core issue in innovative ways. The connections which were developed between tobacco-control and children's charities and with key policy actors—Independent Senator Jillian van Turnhout, who supported the SP legislation was a former Chief Executive of the Irish Children's Rights Alliance—were used to provide evidence to the Oireachtas health committee examining the legislation.

It was evident in the SP debate that policy messages on tobacco control can have additional power when they come from non-tobacco control organisations or people, and particularly when framed in terms of child protection rather than targeting adult smokers. This was also important in defusing attempts by the tobacco industry and others to brand SP as an extreme form of interventionism driven forwards by an ideologically motivated, puritanical anti-smoking lobby. As the respondent cited above commented:

> … you do start to get kind of branded with the kind of health 'Taliban' idea, so if you have other people coming out making slightly different arguments, because it has to be said that the children's charities didn't bring it up with the health issues because it's not relevant to them. They did talk about the marketing it to children and those kinds of things.

This was part of a wider strategy to push back against industry narratives, and reframe the debate in terms more likely to be conducive to the successful introduction of the policy. This involved shifting the emphasis away from industry talking points (e.g. the implications of the measure for trade law and the alleged dangers of contraband and counterfeiting) and emphasising SP as a key measure to protect public health, and particularly children. As the IHF respondent explained:

> So, I suppose that myself and one of the guys in the Cancer Society would have developed a lot of briefing papers. And we also, we were trying to kind of educate people about the issue as well to make them feel comfortable that they could talk on the media about it. So we kind of had regular emails that were updated with what was going on in the world, what's the evidence, and that kind of thing. We also, we commission market research for young people because again, we just wanted to keep shifting away from intellectual property and start talking about what was the real purpose of this legislation, towards children. So we commission market research and that would have been ourselves and the Cancer Society.

NGOs' Coordination with Policy-Makers

As well as the strategic coordination between NGOs in support of SP, there was also important coordination between the NGO sector and policy-makers, such as Health Minister James Reilly, attempting to ensure the passage of SP into law. This saw the NGOs working on SP having regular meetings with Reilly, who led the passage of the SP legislation. A key role of NGOs was to provide support for ministers, particularly in the form of evidence, which they could use to support the proposed policy and provide a rationale for its introduction. As a respondent from the ICS commented:

> So he [Reilly] announced it, and off he went. Now, from our point of view, what we needed to do – we've sat down and discussed it with the Minister and his people, but what we needed to do then was, we needed to keep up the public campaign to show that this was a) a good idea, and b) that it would work … that there was evidence that it would work.

NGOs played a vital role in providing robust, reliable and timely information to key policy actors involved in the parliamentary debate on SP. One senator explained that she relied extensively on evidence supplied to her by the IHF and ICS:

> And for me they did superb research. And we have very busy schedules here, so if I had any questions I'd be able to fling them over to them and they'd go off or they'd cite to me a report to look at, or look at page five on this report, I think that's the information you're seeking.

Given the novelty of the policy, only recently introduced in Australia, firm real-world evidence of the effectiveness of SP was limited at that stage. Consequently, the Irish government relied on research undertaken by the ICS to demonstrate the effectiveness of the policy and widespread public support for it in Ireland:

> One thing we did was, we did some – we produced a report – we got a market research company to do work with teenagers, in particular, on their response to brands, and particularly on their response to tobacco branding. And, so we produced that report […]. They wanted evidence. So they were thrilled when we did the market research. They used that up, down, in out and all around. They quoted that extensively.

Support for the government from the NGO sector, and wider indications of public support for the project, were especially important at specific times in the campaign, at which divisions appeared to emerge between individual ministers and departments within the government. As a respondent from the IHF explained:

> … that was another strategy [of the tobacco industry], to try and isolate [James Reilly, the Health Minister] within the government. I think he was very undermined by our Prime Minister, you know, our Minister of Finance and Minister of Justice meeting with the tobacco industry, and I think the way that process was managed afterwards, he tried to get as much media attention as possible. I think maybe it was a good thing that it happened in one way because it meant then that the government came out very strongly saying we're completely in favour of plain packaging and this is the across the government approach and this is the policy that we want. So, it was in association with him, which it had been up to that point, I think. I think we certainly did help him in providing cover.

In this instance, the close relationship between the Health Ministry and the tobacco-control NGOs meant they were able to use industry attempts to divide the government as the basis for media campaigns to reinforce support for the policy and compel the government to move forwards with their proposed legislation. This built on longer-standing efforts by tobacco-control NGOs to explain the importance of non-engagement with the tobacco industry—in keeping with Ireland's obligations under Article 5.3 of the FCTC—to actors across government. As a respondent from the ICS commented:

> And we have pointed out to the various departments, the – obviously the Department of Finance, the revenue commissioners, and the Department – well, the Department of Health you didn't have to tell them, but, you know, those departments – that they had no business meeting with the tobacco industry, except on purely strict regulatory things. But they say: "Oh, we like to hear from them". I mean, even this year we were in with finance back in… Yeah, last month. September, yeah. And I asked them – I said: "Are you meeting the tobacco industry this year?" And they said: "Oh, yeah we were." And I said: "Well, why – why did you need to meet them?" "We like to hear from them about what's going on." I said but you can't rely on what they tell you.

The dialogue between policy-makers and the NGOs was not unidirectional but worked both ways, with policy advocates benefiting from government briefings. The effectiveness of their campaigning was facilitated by this dialogue with the government and the prior warning they had of policy announcements. This allowed them to have their messaging and props in place in time for announcements to maximise the impact of their work. As a respondent from the ICS commented:

> He [Reilly] announced [the SP policy] publicly [...], but because we were ready for it he told us his plans to announce it then. We were ready for it by way of props for media and all that kind of thing. [...] So, there's no question that without him it wouldn't have happened the way it did.

This approach built on the experience of previous successful campaigns such as the introduction of smoke-free public spaces. As Luke Clancy from the Tobacco Free Research Institute commented:

> I was the Chairman of ASH at the time and we created what was called the Health Alliance and that was bringing together all of the charities who were interested in tobacco control and in conjunction with the Department of Health and with the Health Executive who were going to have to implement it, so that was quite the most directed thing I was involved with and we had an arrangement with the Minister at the time, Micheál Martin, that we would confer, we had weekly meetings which I didn't and he didn't attend. But with our people meeting every week as representatives from the different charities who would review what happened, decide what needed to be done and who needed to do it.

Policy Learning from Australia

The enactment of SP in Australia prior to Ireland meant NGOs in the latter context were able to learn from the experiences of this in the former. As such, we classify this as an example of ***horizontal-consecutive policy learning***. Respondents in Ireland consistently cited the importance of the role played by Australian NGOs, not simply in helping to transfer the *idea* of SP from Australia to Ireland (and other European countries), but in supporting also *the passage of SP legislation* in Ireland, and the work of Irish NGOs in this process. This involved advice on the policy itself and its efficacy, but also on the *tactics* required to counteract the well-organised efforts of TTCs to derail the policy. Mike Daube from Curtin University in Australia, who played an important role in the policy debates in Ireland, highlighted the ease with which NGOs are able to share information, learn from each other and coordinate activities internationally, especially where there is a shared language:

> First of all, from our side, [...] we're pretty well coordinated internationally in tobacco as well. Now we've got our – you know, with thanks to the wonders of email and whatever else, we talk to each other, we link in well with each other. So the moment that the Irish government was going to come out there, they were able to get their briefings, they were able to get – they can just – if you're in Dublin, you can get a superb briefing from [the Cancer Council of Victoria], just as quickly as I can from Perth.

Another actor seconded this and highlighted the importance of technology in facilitating these international NGO networks:

> [There is] a Facebook group of about 2,000 tobacco-control people where we share lots of information and through there people are asking questions and networking and so we stay really connected. I feel like the global tobacco-control community is really well connected, like people know each other quite well, they know who to go to for certain information and they know who's helpful and things like this [...].

Engagement in Irish processes was pro-active on the part of Australian public health actors, and reflected the important role which Canadian public health actors had played in Australian processes, sharing their experiences of unsuccessful attempts to introduce SP there in the 1990s. However, the engagement and coordination between NGOs in Australia and Ireland was also a response to tobacco industry moves to bring in their own allies to speak to the relevance of the Australian case, highlighting industry-favourable arguments against SP. As a respondent from the ICS commented:

> They decided to ship in people from Australia as well. So you have guys from Australian, I think it was the Australian Retailers Association, I don't know, who magically appeared on the radio in Dublin talking about how plain packaging had such an awful effect on Australian business, etc. Never made it clear about who paid for his flights, how did he get here even though we've asked that many times. But they would just magically appear on the media here to talk about the Australian effect. Now we counteract that by

> getting Professor Mike Daube who is from Curtin University to come too. He actually offered himself to come to Ireland to talk about it. So we can't say too much because we got an Australian onto our radio session. Jonathan [Liberman; from the McCabe Centre for Law and Cancer] came at the very, very beginning. […] But yeah no I have to say that what we found very beneficial from our point of view was the Australian input and so we would have very, very strong relationships with not only Jonathan but also Kylie Lindorff [of the Cancer Council Victoria] there as well who would be very keen to know what we're doing and very keen to help out in whatever way that they can. And that was really, really important. I get a phone call from Mike Daube the day of the Parliament, the Parliament passed plain packaging because he was so delighted around like ten, half ten at night to say oh I'm delighted. So from that point of view the Australian influence was really, really beneficial to us as well.

The response to developments in Ireland from the Australian academic and public health communities was extensive and on-going, with key actors highly committed to seeing the passage of SP through in another policy setting, and an EU member state. This reflects the belief on the part of key actors that, while the internal coordination activities between NGOs could be managed at distance, even as great as those between Australia and Ireland, policy-influencing activities and media activities were more effective when undertaken face-to-face or with a physical presence in the policy domain itself. As Mike Daube commented, this made the frequent visits by Australian colleagues of vital importance to the Irish cause:

> I think a personal presence matters too. It's important that you're actually there and that you can talk to the Minister, who can ask you those questions or whatever else, and the media can interview you. But the linkages, just getting information through, are hugely important.

Another Australian public health actor added that the presence of external voices in media debates could be especially important in delivering messages to politicians and the media:

> It's the same everywhere, you bring in an expert from another country he would say exactly the same thing you would say, but for some reason they'd take it – it would mean more to the media if someone from a different country says it. So [the Australian expert] was really valuable in that sort of early push as well.

The extent of Australian engagement reflects also the fact that, until this point, Australia had cut a lone furrow in pursuing SP. The transfer of this policy to another jurisdiction provided a further form of vindication for the policy developments there, and an additional defence against industry criticisms of the policy. From being an outlier, Australia began to assume the position of policy innovator and a strong normative force supporting the development of public health globally. Conversely, were the policy to be rejected in Ireland or be found to contravene some international norms or agreements in the process, then this would have potential ramifications for Australia. The policy process does not end with the passage of legislation; the implementation and evaluation phases are of vital importance, with industry actors looking to shape these in an attempt to discredit, and thus water down or even repeal unfavourable measures. Mike Daube identified "a clear strategy to undermine the outcomes of plain packaging in Australia" on the part of the industry. The passage of similar measures beyond Australia would signify a shift in the perception of SP amongst policy-makers, advocates and the public from experiment to accepted tobacco-control norm. As Mike Daube elaborated:

> So okay, Australia was the first. But we're still – not just geographically – we're still a small country on the other side of the world, and once it had been done somewhere here, [...] then I think it was getting close – I mean, not game over, but it was – then it was going to spread.

A respondent from the IHF also identified this as a key aspect of the Australian NGOs' motivation to give such strong support to the debate in Ireland:

> I mean, I think it has to be said that all of us were like, they're brilliant that they went ahead first but they were also very concerned [...] that if Ireland was to go ahead or we were to fail in introducing the policy that would not be good for Australia. You know, I think they wanted to help us out of the goodness of their hearts but there was also, they kind of needed us to do all of that, I think.

There was also an awareness amongst Australian NGOs that perceptions of the policy there could be shaped by debates in Ireland. Given the increasingly globalised nature of policy discourses (at least in relationship to global health issues such as tobacco control) and linguistic and cultural connections which exist between Ireland, Australia and the UK, there was an awareness amongst Australian actors that misinformation spread by the tobacco industry in the debates in Europe may filter though to domestic audiences or be used by the industry there. As the IHF respondent cited above commented, the desire to ensure accurate representation of the policy situation in Australia was a key motivator for their engagement in Ireland:

> And I suppose they knew also that Australia is going to be discussed a lot in Ireland. It's going to be discussed a lot in the UK. And that was the case. I mean, they were constantly having to battle what was being *said* about what was happening in Australia versus what was [actually] happening in Australia.

The importance of SP being adopted, or at least not rejected, elsewhere is reflected also in the engagement by Australian policy-makers in Ireland alongside scholars and civil society actors. As one public health actor commented:

> And there were many contacts made, and they've been incredibly helpful. I mean incredibly helpful. They really were, right along the way, both from the Department of Health and from the charities as well, you know, Cancer Victoria being the main one really.

Australian advocates, who had established relationships with the Irish Ministry of Health, were enlisted to sell the policy to other sectors of government, which may have had reservations about it. As a respondent from the ICS explained:

> So, Jonathan [Liberman] had come over, and he was going to be in London for the McCabe Law Centre for business there, and so he popped over to speak at a conference, and of course he was speaking on plain packaging. And at the same time, because the [Health] Minister [Reilly] had clearly been working on it behind the scenes, Jonathan met some people from the attorney general's office, and from the Department of Health to advise them on basically what had really happened, and the things to watch out for in here. And interestingly one of the things he said was the first thing the tobacco industry will do is they will buy up, basically, most of the big law firms or all the big law firms in Dublin, because there was definitely going to be a legal case. And this would be by way of robbing the government of the best legal brains in the city.

Developing Effective Strategies

Contacts between the Irish NGOs and colleagues in Australia were focused on the development of an effective advocacy strategy to support the enactment of SP, drawing on the experience of the prior legislative process in Australia. As a respondent from the IHF commented, this led to significant exchange of ideas and resources:

> We did talk to our colleagues in Australia and some, a few of the kind of people who had worked in NGOs over there were over here for different conferences and stuff like that, and we had meetings with them to discuss kind of what were the strategies that had worked in Australia, you know. […]. We approached them but […] there was a constant kind of flow of emails and evidence coming back and forth.

This was reflected in comments from a respondent involved in the policy debates in Australia and in sharing experiences of this with colleagues in Ireland:

> … our big hope was that, you know, by documenting that sort of advocacy process and chain that happened here and the different perspectives of people that that would help other countries to sort of be prepared for the fight. The other thing […] when plain packaging was announced, that it was going ahead, was documenting the arguments against it.

This gave Irish actors prior warning of industry arguments and experience of the best ways to respond to these. For example, the decision to focus on the youth aspect of the policy and frame it as a children's rights issue was informed by experiences in Australia and the guidance received from policy actors there. As the IHF respondent explains:

> So from talking to colleagues in Australia, like, they gave us really good pointers and what they felt we should do. And one of the things they felt was that we really need to bring the children's element to the fore. They said that was what really resonated, like, not just in the policy field but in the media field in Australia. And I suppose in terms of tobacco we hadn't really done that before. You know, we kind of had worked from a health sector approach. So we approached then the kind of the big children's health organisations in Ireland which would be Barnardo's, Children's Rights Alliance, and the Irish Society for the Prevention of Cruelty Against Children.

> [...] And what they said, what our colleagues in Australia said, is certainly what we found. It was when we had different voices talking about the issue, like, people to a certain extent are sick of myself or [...] the Cancer Society talking about tobacco issues. But if they hear, you know, [...] the CEO of Barnardo's, who is considered, you know, he's kind of the opinion-maker of Barnardo's, and if he starts to talk about this issue then people tend to start to take it more seriously because I suppose it's different.

This was reflected by respondents in Australia, who emphasised the important role collaborations with domestic actors outside of tobacco control had played in debates there.

Australian actors were also integral in the decision to reframe the Irish debate to being about 'standardised' rather than 'plain' packaging, which, as discussed previously, was of vital importance in countering potential misperceptions amongst the public that it involved the removal of graphic warnings:

> The other thing that the Australians had said to us that they felt it was good to try and frame the issue in terms of standardised instead of plain packaging. They said they had fallen into a little bit of an issue because, plain packaging, people obviously think about the white box. And that's what the industry had kind of portrayed in all of the advertising. Whereas obviously it's not a white box. It's actually quite a stark image that are on the boxes. So that was really helpful.

Connections Between Public Health Actors in the UK and Ireland

Policy debates in the UK and Ireland developed largely in parallel in the wake of developments in Australia. Therefore, we define the dynamics of connections between public health actors in these two settings as *horizontal-concurrent policy learning*. Australian NGOs and public health actors were also active in UK debates offering similar forms of support to tobacco-control bodies advocating SP there: sharing experiences and insights, and appearing in the media. The relative size of the market compared to either Australia or Ireland, and the importance of the UK as a global health actor, meant the dynamics of the policy debate were different in the UK. As Mike Daube commented, the stakes were much higher for the industry in the UK, and this was reflected in the vehemence of their lobbying campaigns:

> Yeah, I think the lobbying in – and this is no disrespect, or not to diminish what [Irish Health Minister] Reilly and the others did – I think it was tougher here. You've got the big companies that are based here, that are at home here, they're still influential here.
>
> [...] so I think the UK really mattered. And the industry knows that for some reason, other countries still look to the UK as a leader in health and so on. And so I think that's why the UK was really important, and they put everything they could into it.

This is not to underplay the importance of Ireland as a policy innovator on SP, especially when seen within the EU context and the implications the Irish case would have for the wider European market. As Mike Daube continued:

> [...] for the industry, one country's bad enough. Once an EU country had gone, then they were really on their back foot.

The importance of the European dimension is of vital importance in understanding the relationship between the SP debates in Ireland and the UK. An almost symbiotic relationship emerged between the two countries on this issue as the policy debates emerged alongside each other. This manifested itself in a degree of competition between Ireland and the UK to be the first country in Europe to enact the measure, and reinforced Ireland's position as a public health leader in Europe. This desire to be first ended up driving policy forwards in both settings. As an Irish public health actor commented:

> I mean it's [Minister Reilly's] legacy because what he has, you could say it's the first country in EU to bring forward [and enact SP], and granted we did it by a day or whatever. [...] and I'd have been in constant contact with colleagues in the UK, in ASH UK [Action on Smoking and Health UK] and in the Department of Health, who wouldn't have used the Ireland situation very well and says, lads, we can't be second again. And that was used in the UK and it suits us all – those of us in tobacco control, keep this going lads. You know, keep them moving it on. Drive them on. And that's exactly what happened, and then they did drive it on.

Whilst Ireland demonstrated political commitment to SP, the UK, as a far larger polity, possessed significantly greater resources in the health and NGO sectors, which could be marshalled in support of such a controversial measure, notwithstanding the redoubled industry efforts to oppose its introduction in the larger market. As is evident also from the preceding quotation, Ireland enjoyed significant support from governmental and NGO actors in the UK. The Irish government also drew on expertise and advice from leading trade layers in the far larger UK legal services market. Despite explicit recognition within the TPD that member states are able to move beyond the minimum requirements of the Directive to undertake SP, there was a legal challenge undertaken by the industry to the policy in both the UK and Ireland. Irish public health actors interviewed for this study were clear that the existence of parallel policy developments in the UK, and the subsequent linkages of industry litigation against SP in Ireland to the case brought against the UK under EU law, was a big advantage for the Irish government given the extra resources the UK was able to bring to defend the case.

In addition, the UK NGO sector was larger and better resourced than in Ireland, with tobacco-specific bodies such as ASH and large charities engaged on tobacco-related issues, such as Cancer Research UK (CRUK), present in the debate. There is evidence of significant strategic learning between UK and Irish NGOs in the advocacy techniques they employed. For example, the ICS and IHF followed the lead of UK cancer charities to develop tools such as mock packs with the tobacco branding removed to educate decision-makers and the wider public about what was meant by SP and to persuade legislators of its benefits. The mock packs were also important in reframing SP as a child protection issue and were used to demonstrate the power of branding over children's emotional responses to tobacco packs versus standardised variants. As a representative of the ICS, which produced the mock packs in conjunction with the IHF, explained:

> So, what we did was… [Cancer Research UK] had done a very powerful video of kids – of children, school children, looking at packs, and saying: "Oh, they're horrible", you know, or "They're the ones with the horrible pictures? Oh, they're horrible". But looking at the packaging they say: "Oh, that's really nice. That's really nice. That's pink." Pink is in vogue, you know. Pink, pink. And these are girls under the age of 10, you know? So we decided we'd do an Irish version of it – that's one of the things we did. We did an Irish version of it with Irish school kids. And it was very strong, because, of

> course, from a media point of view, from a public point of view, it's one thing to show a British video, but you're far better off showing an Irish video, of course. So we did our Irish version of it.
>
> [...] and that actually got a lot of traction. And the Minister came along and launched it first, and we played the video on the same date, that kind of thing. And the other thing then we did was, we put together an alliance of children's charities, and really – like we did the work – ourselves and the Heart Foundation – we did the work and they came in with us. But it created a much – it created a – from the public's point of view – that there was considerable support among children's charities for this measure.

Whilst the idea for the mock packs came from the UK it was important that Irish NGOs undertook their own versions and produced locally specific supporting materials. This mirrors the insights of the tobacco industry, which tailors global strategies to local contexts. A respondent from the IHF explained the importance of these activities because of the additional power of nationally-specific evidence and materials and the opportunities these provided to policy actors to publicise and explain the measures:

> ... to have something that's very specific to Ireland, because you know, like every nation, Irish people think they're very different to other people, you know. And so we would invite [Minister Reilly] to those types of events to give him as many opportunities as possible to be seen talking about it in a positive way and with children, like, as many photo calls as we could possibly organise with children involved. Because, you know, to try and keep the message for the public that it's about children.

Mock packs were used to highlight that 'plain packaging' did not in fact mean the removal of health warning labels, but simply the logos and colour branding associated with cigarette packs. As a representative of the IHF explained:

> The other thing is that we had mock-ups of the packs made for our specific Irish situation and we carried those around with us all of the time. So when we went and met a politician, you went and put the box down on the table and said, this is what we're talking about, we're not talking about a white box. And again, that was very useful. So this is why it was nice we talked to people about the very same issue. You know, kind of those simple things.

Multi-level Governance and Vertical NGO Networks

As highlighted above, developments on SP in Ireland must be seen in the context of the EU and the TPD. Similarly, it is important to understand the work of domestic NGOs in relation to trans-European and intra-EU networks. This involves a two-way process of engagement between NGOs at the national and supranational levels. Consequently, we categorise this engagement as ***vertical policy learning***, occurring within vertically integrated NGO networks. Given the complex nature of the EU's system of multi-level governance, national-level actors are involved in decision-making at the EU level, whilst EU-level structures shape policy-making at the national level; EU-level policy actors may be conduits for influencing developments within member states; NGOs at the national level may engage EU-level policy-makers directly.

Whilst the Dublin-based NGOs mainly focused on domestic policy debates, they were also aware of, and monitored, EU-level policy developments and sought to influence these, mainly via EU-level affiliates. Asked if they sought to influence policy developments at the EU level, a respondent from the IHF commented:

> Yes. We would. We're a small outfit and we have really a small country so we don't have many MEPs and stuff either. But we're members of the Smoke Free Partnership [SFP] [at the EU-level]. But yeah, we were certainly, like, we did all the, here in Ireland we had consultations on TPD and how it would [work], while it was going through the process.

This was reflected by respondents from the ICS about their policy-influencing work:

> It's principally Dublin-based. Mainly because of the work that comes from the Dublin end is more, you know, is a lot more than the EU level. Now we do have two, at the moment two partnerships with Brussels. One is the association of European Cancer Leagues [ECL] and the other is Smoke Free Partnership. Both of those were members of and signed, you know, signed up and taken part in everything like that. The European role has become increasingly significant as time has gone on.

Brussels-based NGOs such as SFP and ECL were seen to possess EU-specific legal expertise on TPD revision and its implications for SP, and also political insights about likely member-state opposition to SP. As the respondent from the IHF expanded:

> But I suppose they had legal expertise at the European level, that TPD, what was possible, what was necessary to get into the TPD so that countries like Ireland who wanted to go further could go further. And so I suppose they were a real resource for us. And also, in terms of telling us what particular countries, potentially, would have a negative opinion against what Ireland was going to do at that kind of level. Also, like, we'd be a member of the European Heart Network and there's the European Cancer Leagues as well. So they, I mean both those organisations are really interested in the Tobacco Products Directive that was going through, telling us what Commissioners we should be focusing our attention on, whether it was going to the jobs Commissioner at this point or whatever.

However, at certain times Dublin-based NGOs would engage directly in debates occurring in Brussels. This largely took the form of 'lobbying up' from the member-state level to the EU on the TPD, to support the EU-level lobbying by SFP. As a representative of the IHF commented:

> I went over a few times, would have gone to some of the hearings [on the TPD] and would have tried to talk to our MEPs, also Northern Ireland MEPs, some of them which were on the committee writing reports and so on. I mean the thing was I suppose, really all of the Irish MEPs are very much on board for the Tobacco Products Directive, and to talk about the strengths that we wanted to see there. And it was more a case of showing that we were providing them with the information, really, rather than convincing them to change their minds on certain – you know, on other issues, it's different. On this, there was almost, there was relative consensus on this issue across policy-makers, which is unusual.

This was echoed by the respondent from the ICS who saw engagement with the EU level as a two-way process, since Brussels NGOs rely on support and information from their national-level affiliates:

> But since I became involved we've done a lot more trips to Brussels, we've got a lot more contact now, a relationship with MEPs. We have a relationship with the European Commission here in Dublin. So from that point of view it's increasingly, there's increasing work coming from that. So, in terms of the TPD, then, that would've, you know, we would've done a lot of work on that. We feed a lot to the likes of the Smoke Free Partnership and the

> European Cancer Leagues but we also take a lot from them as well, kind of use that to kind of influence Dublin politicians as well because, you know, they will have their own input into the European affairs.

As is evident from this quotation, engagement by national-level NGOs in EU-level policy developments is necessary since member-state governments and other policy actors play key roles in decision-making at the EU level. It is wrong to think of the EU and national levels as separate, hermetically sealed entities within the EU system. What may intuitively be thought of as domestic actors are also EU-level policy actors in different contexts (e.g. national ministers in the Council). The most effective means of influencing decision-making in the Council may thus not be via Brussels-level bodies such as SFP, but via national entities with long-standing relationships with national politicians and ministries, although Brussels-based actors may also engage Permanent Representatives and national delegations to the EU institutions. Likewise, MEPs occupy an ambiguous position between the EU and the member-state levels, being both domestic representatives tied into local, as well as national, political communities, and also part of the Brussels polity. Again, it is domestic (Irish) NGOs which are often the most effective gateway to disseminating information to (Irish) MEPs and convincing them to support EU-level proposals, even though the campaign across national-level NGOs is being coordinated at the EU-level by Brussels-based NGOs. This approach is likely to be crucial given evidence that the tobacco industry itself uses national-level actors to target national politicians as part of a multi-level, multi-jurisdictional lobbying strategy (see Chapter 3 and Hawkins et al. 2018). As a representative of the ICS remarked in relation to their lobbying work on the TPD:

> Well from our perspective we were very much concentrating on what the influence in [the European] Parliament was being at that time. So we were well aware – because of again our relationship with SFP – we were very clear about what the tactics were by the tobacco industry in terms of influencing MEPs. Now having said that because again Ireland has quite a small cohort of MEPs we sought to see if any of them had been influenced by the tobacco industry. We couldn't find any evidence of that purely because they were concentrating on German, UK, French, the big countries as opposed to the Irish. But having said that, you know when you have one tobacco company with 150-odd lobbyists at one time in Parliament lobbying specifically on TPD they're naturally going to come across the guys.

Irish NGOs played a particularly important part in the passage of the TPD, given the vital role played by Ireland in the passage of the Directive during its Presidency of the Council in the first half of 2013. As a respondent from the ICS explained:

> In terms of TPD, [...] the revised TPD was kind of pushed forward in the agenda by the Irish Government when it had the Presidency back in 2013. And because of that it was kind of the onus was almost on the Irish Cancer Society to make sure that we backed up the minister in terms of what he was asking for in TPD. So what we would do in terms of us ourselves, in terms of TPD it was primarily focused on the MEPs themselves. [...] Specifically Irish MEPs. We're quite lucky in terms of being from Ireland as opposed to other EU countries because we've only got eleven MEPs. Which is very small in comparison to the other countries, you know? So we would have developed a relationship with those MEPs, making sure that they were aware that this is something that we took a great interest in and that we would be watching them to see how they would react. So in terms of what we would do then, for example the Smoke Free Partnership would be producing a lot of material that we would then give onto the MEPs [...]. They [the SFP] would have a lot more technical knowledge than we would in terms of, you know, amendments to the TPD, what they were voting on in Brussels and Strasbourg. So we would basically be the conduit from SFP to those Irish MEPs at the same time. So that would be primarily what we would've been doing around TPD.

In terms of influence over the passage of SP legislation in Ireland, respondents from EU-level NGOs played a less significant role than Australian and UK NGOs. This is perhaps unsurprising given the extensive opposition to packaging restrictions within the TPD debates. The resources of EU-level NGOS had been channelled towards the TPD, with perhaps limited capacity available to intervene in domestic policy debates in the recent aftermath of this, when other sources of expertise were available from Australia. In addition, the parallel development of policy debates in the UK meant solidarity for the Irish case, and knowledge transfer between NGOS within the EU, emerged mainly from the UK, which was facing similar efforts by the industry to prevent SP.

Summary

Policy developments in Ireland must be seen in their wider European and global contexts, and understood in terms of the transnational NGO networks that facilitated the adoption of SP. Despite the political leadership shown by the Irish government domestically, and at the EU level during its Presidency of the Council, the trail for SP had been blazed globally by Australia, with a vital role played by public health actors and tobacco-control NGOs in securing the introduction of SP there. Australian NGOs had direct experience of the political challenges of introducing a novel and controversial policy and the tactics employed by TTCs in opposition to this. As such, they offered a potentially vital resource for understanding industry strategies and the arguments TTCs would employ against SP. In addition, they were able to share their experience of the most effective ways to counter industry arguments and develop effective advocacy strategies. Given the deep historical, political and economic ties that exist between Ireland and the UK, policy developments in each setting are often highly interconnected. The concurrent development of legislation introducing SP in both contexts meant that the resources available to NGOs, and even government actors, in the much larger polity across the Irish Sea were a further source of support for Irish NGOs. However, policy influence was not unidirectional. Whilst Irish NGOs may have drawn on the resources of their UK-based counterparts, the commitment to SP in Ireland was vital in securing the political will for the final adoption of the policy in the UK, despite indications this may be dropped by the government in the later stages of the policy process. Irish NGOs are embedded in EU-level networks, but the main influence in this relationship was support provided by domestic actors to policy developments at the EU level in the form of the TPD, rather than support for SP domestically via EU-level networks. The weaker vertical interactions on SP reinforced the importance of horizontal forms of support emanating from Australia and the UK.

Bibliography

Hawkins, B., Holden, C., & Mackinder, S. (2018). A multi-level, multi-jurisdictional strategy: Transnational tobacco companies' attempts to obstruct tobacco packaging restrictions. *Global Public Health*. https://doi.org/10.1080/17441692.2018.1446997.

CHAPTER 6

Discussion and Conclusion

Abstract This chapter discusses the study findings in light of relevant theory on policy transfer and multi-level governance. Three theoretical conclusions are made: (1) public health policies today are often subject to a policy transfer 'web', in which networks of actors involving both policymakers and non-governmental organisations (NGOs) are required to navigate various different jurisdictions and levels of governance in order to ensure that a policy is successfully adopted; (2) transnational corporations have analytically-significant consequences for policy transfer processes and may act intentionally to disrupt such processes; and (3) the activities of transnational corporate actors can shape subsequent transfer processes, as policy-makers and NGOs build relationships and coalitions in an effort to adapt to, and counteract, global corporate political strategies.

Keywords Policy transfer · Multi-level governance · Transnational tobacco companies · Standardised packaging · Plain packaging · EU Tobacco Products Directive

This volume has sought to examine the development of standardised packaging (SP) policy in Europe at both the European Union (EU) and member-state levels, placing developments in Europe within the global context of tobacco-control debates and processes. As the analysis above

B. Hawkins et al., *The Battle for Standardised Cigarette Packaging in Europe*, Palgrave Studies in Public Health Policy Research,
https://doi.org/10.1007/978-3-030-31034-9_6

demonstrates, SP has endured a difficult and contentious journey from policy idea through to implementation, and at the time of writing the battle is far from over. The story of the development of the policy, and the actors that have worked for its implementation, demonstrates the complex political environment that public health advocates must navigate within the EU's system of multi-level governance (MLG). Through a case study of Ireland, and employing the concepts of policy transfer and policy learning, this volume has demonstrated the regional and global significance of national policy debates, and the interconnections between policy debates in different policy-making jurisdictions. This chapter relates the empirical analysis presented in Chapters 3–5 to the literature on MLG and policy transfer presented in Chapter 2. It seeks to explain tobacco industry strategy in opposing SP in Europe, to prevent policy 'contagion' across different policy-making jurisdictions and at different levels of governance, and the responses of policy-makers and non-governmental organisations (NGOs) to this corporate activity.

The chapter is structured as follows. The following section discusses the key role of Australia as a policy innovator on SP and its implications for policy development in Europe and beyond. The Australian case demonstrates the understanding which transnational tobacco companies (TTCs) had of the potential for policy transfer to other jurisdictions, were SP to be successfully adopted there, and the vehemence with which they therefore sought to oppose the policy. The second section explores the theoretical implications of the battle over the packaging requirements included within the 2014 EU Tobacco Products Directive (TPD), as the TTCs attempted to disrupt the potential of the EU to become a 'massive transfer platform' (Radaelli 2000). The third section looks at the subsequent policy battle in Ireland. It examines the interconnections between policy debates and policy actors in Ireland, Australia and the UK in light of the policy transfer literature, and how TTCs' tactics affected those relationships. The final section elaborates three theoretical conclusions which contribute to our understanding of policy transfer: (1) public health policies today are often subject to a policy transfer 'web', in which networks of actors, including both policy-makers and NGOs, are required to navigate different levels of governance and jurisdictions in order to ensure that a policy is successfully adopted; (2) transnational corporations have analytically-significant consequences for policy transfer processes and may act intentionally to disrupt such processes; and (3) the activities of transnational corporate actors can shape subsequent policy transfer processes, as policy-makers and NGOs build relationships and coalitions in an effort to counteract corporate political strategies designed to prevent the adoption of public policies that run counter to their narrow corporate interests.

Australia as Policy Leader

As the first country in the world to adopt SP, Australia was subject to a barrage of well-coordinated activities by TTCs in an attempt to overturn the policy. This activity is consistent with other studies of TTC political behaviour, which demonstrate continuing aggressive political behaviour by TTCs over a number of decades (Hurt et al. 2009; Holden and Lee 2009; Smith et al. 2013; Savell et al. 2014). Previous studies have shown that TTCs were concerned not only with the impact of SP on sales in any particular jurisdiction, but with the potential for the policy idea to spread to other jurisdictions and become more widely adopted (Jarman 2015; Hawkins et al. 2018). Corporate actors are somewhat neglected in the policy transfer literature, with theoretical insights focused predominantly on the activities of policy-makers and advocates (see Chapter 2). However, the analysis presented above demonstrates that transnational corporations can be important actors within policy transfer processes, seeking to disrupt and prevent the diffusion of policy ideas and block successful transfer. Their substantial economic resources mean they are formidable opponents for both governments and NGOs seeking to implement or advocate for policy measures in the public interest.

As Australia sought to implement SP, TTCs initiated highly sophisticated, globally-coordinated political strategies to oppose the policy, which included lobbying and policy-influencing strategies, the use of third parties and multiple, concurrent legal challenges under different bodies of law (including the Australian constitution, the Australia–Hong Kong Bilateral Investment Treaty [BIT] and World Trade Organization [WTO] law) in an attempt to prevent or delay the introduction of SP (Hawkins and Holden 2016; Hawkins et al. 2018). The strength of their response to the introduction of SP at the state level suggests that their concerns went beyond the economic impact that the legislation could have on the Australian market alone. Rather, they demonstrated a significant concern that the implementation of SP in Australia could establish the principle that this was an effective form of policy intervention, compatible with international trade law and other commitments, and could trigger 'policy contagion' to other policy contexts, including their most important and profitable markets. Preventing policy transfer was therefore a key objective of TTCs in Australia. Due to their economic and political power, corporate actors can shape, delay and potentially prevent the implementation of a policy that they consider to be against their interests. Consequently, they should be an important analytical focus within policy transfer scholarship, and are underrepresented in the existing literature.

While Australia was targeted by the TTCs as the first state-level jurisdiction to implement SP, it was nevertheless a relatively small and declining tobacco market. The introduction of SP in the much larger EU market represented a significantly greater economic threat to the tobacco industry, given its population of over 500 million high-income consumers, highly evolved supranational governance structures that maintain coercive and normative power, and policy networks that could accelerate policy transfer. Moreover, the potential for policy adoption at the EU level and at the member-state level meant there were multiple potential routes through which policy transfer could occur, with the likelihood that adoption in one member state, if deemed compatible with EU law, would rapidly spread to others.

Strengthened Packaging Requirements in the EU: The Tobacco Products Directive

Studies of TTCs' attempts to oppose SP in Australia underline the way in which they implemented a multi-level strategy to challenge SP simultaneously on multiple fronts and at different levels of governance (Chapman and Freeman 2014; Hawkins and Holden 2016; Hawkins et al. 2018). These revealed the importance of 'venue-shifting' to direct policy decisions to those contexts in which a favourable outcome for the industry was most likely. Whilst in the Australian case this involved national law, as well as bilateral and global-level regimes, the existence of the EU as a strong regional institution added a further layer of complexity to policy-making in Europe. The EU represented a double-edged sword for TTCs. The capacity of the EU to introduce effective and enforceable tobacco-control measures under the auspices of single-market law represented an additional mechanism through which SP (or other packaging requirements) could be introduced across the twenty-eight member states, and thus posed an additional threat to tobacco companies. Even where collective action at the EU level could be avoided (as was the case with SP in the TPD), the close political ties and high levels of policy coordination that exist between EU member states meant that once a policy idea such as SP came onto the agenda in one member state, it had the potential to spread rapidly to others. The EU's role as a 'massive transfer platform' (Radaelli 2000) and a 'supranational idea hopper' (Bomberg and Peterson 2000) could significantly speed up policy contagion. At the same time, the highly developed legal structures within the EU, and the emphasis afforded to 'market-making' functions within its treaties, provided a further avenue through which SP at the EU level and within member states could be challenged (Holden and Hawkins 2017).

Given the size of the market, and the potential for the policy to be implemented at once across the twenty-eight member states, the EU was a key battleground for TTCs in the fight against SP. The timing of the TPD revision had both positive and negative aspects for the TTCs. Working to their disadvantage was the fact that the rotating Presidency of the Council was held by Ireland in the first semester of 2013—a key stage in the conclusion of the TPD. The Irish Government and Health Minister James Reilly held a strong political commitment to the successful conclusion of the TPD negotiations.

However, there were several structural factors within the EU institutional architecture that worked in the TTCs' favour. The political timetables in the EU, the European Parliament election scheduled for early 2014, and the subsequent appointment of a new Commission, meant that delaying the TPD—a key aspect of the industry's strategy—could result in the legislation failing to pass before the dissolution of Parliament, necessitating the reintroduction of the TPD by a new Commission and its approval by a newly constituted European Parliament (EP) which might have a very different political outlook and set of priorities. Moreover, the governments of Lithuania (second semester 2013) and Greece (first semester 2014), who would succeed Ireland in the Council Presidency, were considered to have weaker positions on tobacco control and consequently, advocates feared, may not have had the political determination to conclude agreement on such a controversial portfolio. The complex institutional structure of the EU provided further advantages for TTCs, as the conflicting mandates and priorities of different policy actors provided opportunities to play interests off against each other. This approach has been identified in other policy areas, including studies of environmental policy making in the EU (e.g. Jordan et al. 2003).

The analysis presented in this volume demonstrates that the TTCs developed a sophisticated, coordinated strategy that sought to exploit these advantages and stymie development of the TPD at every step of the policy-making process. TTCs employed evolving strategies at the various different stages of the policy process and via multiple points of access, demonstrating their ability to exploit the complexities of the EU's institutional architecture and disrupt the progression of policies through several different approaches. They lobbied every institution within the EU legislative process—the Commission, the Council and the Parliament—and initiated legal challenges to the TPD under EU law once it had been adopted.

In the policy development stage they targeted the Commission, seeking to undermine the leading Directorate General (DG) on the TPD, DG SANCO, by attempting to venue-shift to other DGs that were more favourable to their agenda and to challenge the narrative being developed in DG SANCO. Reflecting Baumgartner and Jones' (1991) analysis that venue-shifting requires changing the 'policy image', TTCs attempted to reframe the debate in economic terms, with a specific focus on jobs and taxes; important considerations for member states that had economic interests associated with the tobacco industry (cigarette production, packaging manufacture, etc.), and therefore a powerful counter-narrative to the considerations about public health underpinning SP. The flooding of the inter-services consultation with responses and attempts to use committees other than ENVI to influence the TPD in the EP, demonstrate further the TTCs' intricate understanding of EU policy processes.

TTCs' efforts at agenda setting were partially successful. They appear to have prevented the adoption of SP at the EU level early in the Commission's processes and managed to ensure that the minimum requirements for packaging were significantly watered down (Costa et al. 2014; Peeters et al. 2015). In short, despite the stipulation in Article 5.3 of the Framework Convention on Tobacco Control (FCTC) that governments should take measures to protect health policy from 'commercial and other vested interests of the tobacco industry' (WHO 2003), the TTCs had successfully disrupted the potential of the EU to disperse SP throughout Europe (see Radaelli 2000). This demonstrates the point that changes in ideas alone are insufficient as an explanatory theory of policy change. Despite the idea of SP spreading from Australia to Europe, this was not enough to ensure the adoption of SP at the EU level. Rather, institutional structures, political processes, vested interests, competing policy priorities and relationships between actors are of vital importance in explaining policy change or stasis.

Of particular importance is the presence of *coercion* and the power relationships between key policy actors. As Dobbin et al. (2007) point out, coercion theory focuses most obviously on mechanisms of policy control, such as conditionality, emanating from organisations such as the World Bank or the International Monetary Fund (IMF). However, political scientists, such as Stone (2007) and Gleditsch and Ward (2006), also argue that policy leadership and hegemonic ideas can be 'soft' forms of coercion. These theories are united by a focus on the impact of influences or ideas from *external* sources on the policy-making process. In this instance, the TTCs challenged the EU's normative power, pursuing a strategy to promote a counter-idea around economic and jobs considerations, which had the potential to weaken the power of the idea of SP.

The development of the TPD was not an outright victory for the TTCs, however. Although SP did not become part of the TPD, and the labelling requirements that were finally adopted were significantly watered down from the original proposals, these represented a significant advance on the previous minimum packaging requirements. Moreover, by including an explicit recognition that member states could proceed with SP at the national level, the TPD offered both a clear normative endorsement of these measures for governments and potential cover from subsequent legal challenges by the tobacco industry. This provided an important legal 'springboard' for policy action by Ireland and other member states.

Ireland

By the time the TPD was adopted, measures to implement SP in Ireland were already in train. Ireland had been long recognised as a leader in the area of tobacco control both within Europe and globally. Despite the political commitment for SP evident in Ireland, however, the government and public health advocates faced a significant challenge in implementing the policy from TTCs opposed to its introduction. The transfer of the policy idea of SP from Australia to Ireland was only the first stage in a protracted political and legal battle for its realisation. This had to be supplemented by significant cooperation and policy learning between NGOs and advocates in Ireland and Australia, with the former drawing on the experience of, and employing the strategies developed by, those in the latter to secure the policy's successful adoption and implementation.

Policy Learning Across Jurisdictions

Irish public health advocates turned to those in Australia for guidance on how to manage the policy-making process. Irish actors sought guidance from Australian colleagues on how to get SP successfully through the legislative process and into implementation. Central to this process was the role played by transnational NGO networks engaged in what we have termed here *horizontal-consecutive policy learning*. This builds on Evans and Davies' (1999) model of policy transfer, which traces the linear progression of a policy from 'exporter' to 'importer' jurisdictions. They draw on the literature on policy networks and epistemic communities to analyse how policy-makers 'acquire and utilize knowledge' (Evans and Davies 1999, 376; see Chapter 2). In the case of SP, the 'information feeder network' and 'transfer network' were not only the Australian policy-makers who contributed to the successful implementation of the policy there, but also the tobacco-control NGOs who played a key role in that implementation. In addition to their relationship with Australian actors, Irish actors also created a transfer pathway with the UK, which we have termed *horizontal-concurrent policy learning*. As the UK was exploring the possibility of SP at the same time as Ireland, there were exchanges of information and important crossover points between the policy processes. The far larger political community and resource base in the UK meant that both sides in the Irish debate (TTCs and tobacco-control NGOs) drew on the resources available there in an attempt to influence the domestic policy process. Again, these transfer relationships not only facilitated discussion and knowledge exchange about how to develop the policy, they were also used to share knowledge on how to combat the activities of the TTCs so as to see the policy through to successful implementation.

Transnational Corporations as Strategic Actors

As discussed previously, Ireland was known to be a 'leader' in tobacco control, having led the charge in Europe for smoke-free public spaces in 2004, and had also been influential in the fight for the revision of the TPD in the EU. Its previous role as a policy 'exporter' was a particular threat to the TTCs, who feared 'policy contagion' within the EU, and pursued a coordinated, multi-faceted strategy to prevent the implementation of SP in Ireland. The political and economic context in Ireland at the time of the SP debates (see Chapter 4) was a key structural factor, which offered TTCs new avenues and opportunities to seek to influence the Irish government at a time of great vulnerability. The post-2008 economic crisis faced by Ireland increased the TTCs' capacity for economic coercion, and Ireland's integration in the global economy, including its dependence on foreign direct investment (FDI) from the US, offered additional 'points of attack' and channels of engagement with the Irish government. The close relationships that TTCs maintained with important political actors and institutions in the US—for example congressional representatives from tobacco-growing states—offered a bilateral channel of influence. The TTCs' long-standing strategy of attempting to frame tobacco control debates in terms of economic considerations and intellectual property (IP) rights, versus health (Savell et al. 2014; MacKenzie et al. 2018), was particularly pertinent in the context of the economic crisis. Similarly, Ireland's membership of the EU, and its reliance on EU economic assistance following the crisis, offered supranational channels of influence which TTCs sought to exploit, by encouraging supportive member states and other actors within EU institutions (e.g. economic and trade-focused DGs within the Commission) to exert political pressure on Ireland.

In addition to reframing the debate as one of economic consequences and IP, they promoted the idea that SP would lead to increased illicit trade and would damage the high street in an attempt to counter the public health arguments of tobacco-control actors, precisely as they had done in Australia. In terms of Evans and Davies' (1999) model of policy transfer, TTCs targeted every stage of the transfer process between Ireland and Australia (see Chapter 2). Within these stages, transfer agents were identified, and information feeder networks and transfer networks were built. Within this process, evidence from Australia was garnered, shared, evaluated and mobilised by tobacco-control advocates and policy-makers, while TTCs sought to undermine this evidence and the agents that provided it.

Working to the TTCs' advantage was the fact that SP had only very recently been enacted in Australia, so there was limited evidence emerging from that country that could affirm the policy's efficacy as a tobacco-control measure. TTCs, therefore, attempted to challenge the evidence from Australia provided by the transfer network and cited by policy advocates in support of the measures in Ireland. Furthermore, the limited evidence base allowed the industry to make unsubstantiated claims about the lack of effectiveness and the adverse consequences of the policy (e.g. increased illicit trade). The TTCs, therefore, developed their own transfer relationships between Australia and Ireland at this point, creating an alternative 'evidence' base to challenge SP and shipping in pro-tobacco advocates from Australia in order to disparage the policy through media and policy channels.

The final tactic that the TTCs used to disrupt the transfer of SP and contain the policy 'contagion' were legal challenges. This started with threats of legal action to the Irish government early in the policy process, which again drew parallels with the on-going experience of the Australian government. Letters were sent by TTCs to the Irish government outlining their intent to oppose the policy through the courts, and emphasising the potential consequences to an already struggling Irish economy.

The policy transfer literature does not focus explicitly on the consequences of legal challenges on the policy transfer process, although it does draw on Kingdon's (1984) work on agenda setting to address more general considerations about the *political* feasibility of the transfer of particular policies from one jurisdiction to another. SP already had political feasibility in Ireland; there was a high degree of public support for the policy. The tactics of the TTCs, however, shifted the venue in which the success or otherwise of the policy would be determined from the political sphere to the legal sphere. This points to an aspect of the policy process that has been under-analysed within the policy transfer literature; the potential ability to block or delay the actual implementation of the policy through its contestation by non-state actors.

This chapter and the analysis presented above demonstrate the potential for the wielding of coercive power by transnational corporations; various forms of legal redress provide important mechanisms for the realisation of this coercive power. The potential for concurrent legal challenges at multiple levels, through both domestic courts and through supranational channels via the WTO, BITs or the EU legal architecture presented myriad opportunities for TTCs to employ this coercive power, as both the Australian and European experience of SP demonstrates (Hawkins and Holden 2016; Hawkins et al. 2018). In the Irish context specifically, JTI began proceedings in the Irish commercial courts, arguing that as an EU member state Ireland could not unilaterally impose SP, as it went beyond the stipulations of the TPD and ran counter to EU single-market law. The substantive points of law were decided in a parallel case referred to the CJEU via the English courts and the industry's action failed.

The TTCs' tactics presented a potentially significant problem for policymakers and advocates in Ireland. This highlights a gap in the policy transfer literature, relating to the potential for non-state actors to contest policy and attempt to disrupt the transfer process to prevent policy 'contagion'. The existing literature engages with the role of non-state actors within the policy transfer process, but focuses largely on their role as transfer *facilitators*; civil society actors coalescing around a policy idea and knowledge base. Dolowitz and Marsh (1996) identified this group as including political consultants, but this was broadened by Dunlop (2009) and Stone (2004, 2012) to include a wider array of actors such as NGOs, think tanks and philanthropic organisations. Corporate actors are considered in passing within these studies in terms of their relationship to these other actors; for example, Hudson and Lowe (2009) identify how corporate actors use organisations such as think tanks to forward their agendas. Corporations are also mentioned in 'opposition' to policies in situations where policy advocates (who remain the analytical focus) have coalesced against them (Hudson and Lowe 2009). However, in these analyses, the impact of the corporation on the transfer process is not considered as a primary analytical focus.

Against this, the analysis in the current volume suggests that corporate actors can be a key influence on policy-making and, therefore, policy transfer processes. In cases such as tobacco packaging, in which the commercial interests of powerful transnational corporations are threatened by proposed regulations, corporate actors pro-actively seek to challenge and undermine the transfer process to prevent policy 'contagion' from one domain to another. This is a logical extension of wider corporate political strategies, which seek to secure political outcomes favourable to their interests. A bias in the literature towards *successful* instances of transfer may be an important factor in explaining the under-representation of corporate actors in existing studies, in that examples where transnational corporate actors have been successful in disrupting policy transfer may be less visible and are less amenable to study, in the same way that policy stasis, or the absence of policy change, more generally proves elusive to study. This point becomes clearer in light of Dolowitz and Marsh's (1996, 2000) framework for the analysis of policy transfer and, more specifically, their analysis of factors which restrict or facilitate policy transfer processes, and the ways in which the process of policy transfer is related to policy 'success' or policy 'failure' (see Chapter 2). Dolowitz and Marsh's (1996, 2000) responses to these questions focus on issues of policy complexity, institutional context and information deficits; the fact that actors may enter the transfer process with the explicit objective of *preventing* the policy transfer to protect their own interests is not considered within this framework.

The Evolution of Policy Learning Between Ireland, Australia and the UK

The policy transfer relationship between Australia and Ireland, facilitated through transnational NGO networks, did not end with the entry of SP onto the policy agenda in Dublin. Tobacco-control advocates in Ireland also turned to Australia for ideas, advice and expertise throughout the policy process, including on the ways in which they could support the adoption and implementation of the policy *in the face of TTC opposition* throughout the legislative and implementation processes. As the interviews demonstrate, this changed the nature and the context of the policy transfer process itself; the TTCs changed the actions of the agents involved in the process and the relationship between them. The original transfer agents and contributors to what Evans and Davies (1999) term the 'information feeder network' were Australian tobacco-control NGOs. However, these tobacco-control NGOs were also, in Evans and Davies' (1999) terms, acting as not only the transfer agents, but also the information network and the knowledge network. The work of Diane Stone (2004, 2012) on non-state actors, and specifically NGOs, is also pertinent here, since the 'transnationalisation' of policy through non-state actors is again evident. Australian NGOs and policy-makers shared their experience and knowledge with Irish policy-makers and NGOs who were working in an advocacy capacity. These NGOs therefore became the 'epistemic community' for *strategies* related to policy adoption and implementation (as opposed to the initial idea) and the line was blurred between those acting in a 'knowledge' capacity and an 'advocacy' capacity.

As we have seen, the role soon evolved into one that included sharing information and advice on how to protect the policy from industry attack. The 'knowledge network' gave prior warnings as to what the TTCs may do, and what arguments they may deploy, to contest the policy, and shared advice and experience on how to pre-empt, react and respond to the TTCs' tactics and issue framings, including advising the Irish policy community how to use the media to support the policy. These strategies ensured that the information and evidence provided by the knowledge network, limited as it was, was able to overcome the counter-narratives and alternative 'evidence' being promoted by the TTCs. The role of the 'information feeder network' was therefore highly politicised, and much broader than the role presented in much of the policy transfer literature; it addressed not only the content of the policy, but also how to *protect* the policy from those seeking to derail it.

These protection strategies in turn altered the make-up of the advocacy network itself. The TTCs had gone to some lengths to reframe the debate about SP in terms of IP rights, arguing that SP constituted illegal expropriation of their trademarks by the government without compensation. In order to counter this argument, Australian NGOs advised Irish policy-makers and NGOs to broaden the advocacy network of the tobacco-control actors to include advocates from other sectors and to reframe the 'policy image' to include the wider implications of the policy, such as the impact on children. In so doing, policy advocates directly challenged the TTCs' IP rights argument with a rights-based argument of their own. The transfer agents therefore deliberately expanded the advocacy network to include representatives from other lobbies, such as children's societies, in order to develop and build a broader argument, that went beyond the remit of public health, with which to counter the TTCs' narrative. It is important to reiterate that the benefits of policy transfer were not unidirectional, however. The Australian tobacco-control community was keen to support Ireland and the UK in their efforts to implement SP, as their own policy was under attack and the external validation of their policy entrepreneurship, in the form of other countries adopting the policy, would support policy advocates' own efforts to counter TTCs' attempts to undermine and repeal the measure at home. The policy transfer process was therefore used not only as a mechanism to inform colleagues in a new policy setting about the prior experiences of other jurisdictions, it was intentionally developed to ensure the success of the policy in both jurisdictions.

This case of SP in Europe therefore offers several new insights into the policy transfer process, particularly with regard to the role of transnational corporate actors who seek to not only become involved in the transfer process, but to disrupt and undermine it, and to use transfer mechanisms themselves for this purpose. Revisiting Dolowitz and Marsh's (1996) heuristic framework helps emphasise this point, as the questions they forward to establish policy transfer mechanisms reveal several analytical insights not as yet discussed in the literature:

1. *Who are the key actors involved in the policy transfer process?* Although transnational corporations are sometimes mentioned in this regard, the literature tends to focus on the most common agents of policy transfer—elected officials, policy entrepreneurs or experts, political

parties, bureaucrats, advocacy groups and supranational institutions (Dolowitz and Marsh 1996, 2000; Evans 2009). The case analysed in this volume has demonstrated that this question, however, raises another pertinent question—who seeks to *prevent* policy transfer? Transnational corporate actors not only can use transfer mechanisms themselves to forward their own political agendas, but may actively seek to disrupt the transfer processes of other actors. Furthermore, they hold some coercive power, through their economic importance in some countries, through their well-organised political agency and through their ability to exploit legal mechanisms, particularly those at the supranational level. They can therefore be significant actors in the transfer process, in ways not well investigated so far in the literature.

2. *Why engage in policy transfer?* Dolowitz and Marsh (1996, 2000) framed policy transfer in terms of voluntary and coercive mechanisms, the latter being what differentiated it from 'lesson-drawing'. They argued that policy transfer came about inter alia through the dissatisfaction of policy-makers, public unhappiness, perceived policy failure, and uncertainty. This case demonstrates however that a key explanatory factor that consolidated the transfer pathways and their associated networks between Ireland, Australia and the UK was the need to counteract the activities of the TTCs. Relationships between pro-public health policy-makers and NGOs were forged and strengthened in part in order to share tactics and form a coalition that resisted TTCs' strategy of trying to block, amend or delay the policy.
3. *What elements of policy are transferred?* Dolowitz and Marsh (1996, 2000) listed a number of 'hard' policy instruments such as policy goals, policy instruments, institutions and programmes, which others such as Stone (2004, 2012) expanded to include 'softer' elements of policy, such as ideas, ideologies and concepts. In this case we can see that although policy ideas, goals and instruments were transferred, as important were political *strategies and tactics* to ensure that the policy was adopted and carried through to implementation.
4. *From where are policies transferred?* The traditional transfer literature focused predominantly on bilateral transfer between national governments (e.g. Jones and Newburn 2006). As the theory evolved, the 'internationalisation' of the theory saw more of a preoccupation with forces such as globalisation, Europeanisation and multi-level governance, which studied vertical pathways of transfer as well as horizontal pathways. This case importantly demonstrates that one policy had

multiple different potential transfer pathways, which could be concurrent as well as consecutive; SP was blocked at the EU level, but strengthened packaging requirements were nevertheless transferred vertically from the EU's supranational level to set a floor for member states, with the TPD specifically allowing action on SP at the national level; at the same time, several horizontal pathways emerged between Ireland, Australia and the UK to address the implementation of the policy and to counteract the TTCs' contestation. This suggests that for analytical rigour, it is necessary to break down policies into 'component parts' in order to understand the transfer and diffusion of policies in an increasingly globalised world, and to take particular account of the different possible pathways within multi-level systems of governance.

5. *What factors enable and constrain transfer?* The traditional literature focuses on policy complexity as the main constraint to transfer, arguing that policy complexity and embeddedness in wider social and political contexts can impede transfer from one jurisdiction to another (Dolowitz and Marsh 1996, 2000; Evans 2009). The increase in non-state actors and multi-level governance structures through increased globalisation has the potential to uncover further constraints, which Benson and Jordan (2011) argue have not yet been analysed sufficiently in the literature. What is not mentioned, importantly, is *deliberate contestation of the policy and its transfer*. With the omission of transnational corporate actors from the analysis, and the bias in the empirical literature towards 'successful' instances of transfer, an important transfer constraint can be overlooked, i.e. the presence of actors actively trying to prevent transfer—or 'contagion'—occurring when a policy idea goes against their interests.

Conclusion

By applying policy transfer theory to the development of standardised packaging policy, this volume has demonstrated that transnational corporate actors can have a significant impact on the transfer potential and efficacy of public health policies. Three theoretical conclusions can be drawn from this case. The first refers both to the transit of the policy idea itself and to the development of the tactics needed to ensure its adoption. In a globalised world, the potential pathways of transfer are multiple and may be concurrent as well as consecutive. This is particularly true in multi-level polities such as the EU. Furthermore, networks of policy actors engaged in the exchange of ideas, knowledge and tactics may be crucial to the successful adoption of the policy within such multi-level systems. We can conclude, therefore, that the increase in multi-level governance structures creates a complex matrix which transfer networks must navigate, creating policy transfer 'webs' that differ from the bilateral modes of transfer studied in much of the literature.

The second theoretical conclusion relates to the role of transnational corporate actors. Such actors have in general been neglected in the literature, other than as indirect sponsors of think tank research in policy areas where they have a business interest (Hudson and Lowe 2009). While there is certainly evidence of this in this study, a much more direct link to the transfer process is also apparent. We see here that TTCs were ***directly concerned*** with policy transfer—or from their perspective policy 'contagion'. Consequently, their strategies were built around preventing transfer, with some level of success, as seen in their activities surrounding the TPD. Furthermore, these transnational corporate actors have coercive power—their economic weight and political sophistication mean that they can apply pressure both directly and through enlisting other nation states to apply pressure on their behalf. The complex supranational legal architecture of institutions such as the WTO and the EU also provides them several points of potential coercion through legal threats and actions. Additionally, transnational corporate actors may not only seek to disrupt the transfer process, they can also create their own transfer pathways—in this case, mirroring the transfer relationship between Irish and Australian NGOs to transport members of their own epistemic network (which supports the counter-idea of the negative impacts of SP) from Australia to Ireland.

This integration of transnational corporate actors within the policy transfer process has several analytical consequences. Their omission from the literature means that a significant global source of power is missing from current theory. The consequences of their activities include the disruption or prevention of transfer, which may result in transfer failure—an important aspect of analysis, as Dolowitz and Marsh's (1996, 2000) heuristic framework demonstrates. Their activities could also be a cause of variations in the implementation of policies, or the timing of their adoption, which may also be influenced by structural factors such as a country's perceived economic reliance on an industry, or historical factors that facilitate or constrain an industry's coercive power.

Another consequence of transnational corporate actors' activities within the transfer process relates to our third theoretical conclusion, which addresses the transfer pathways that emerged in response to TTCs' activities. While there is some policy transfer literature that refers to the exchange of political tactics (e.g. Pierson and Castles 2002), this example differs from this sub-literature in two ways. The first is that, in this example, the tactical exchange is not about defeating domestic political opponents; rather, it is about how to combat policy opponents that are active *across* jurisdictions in trying to prevent the transfer process. Second, the transfer pathways of policy-maker and NGO networks became part of a political strategy to secure the success of the policy. Australian advocates deliberately shared their experience with Ireland and the UK not only to help them in their battle with the TTCs, but also because having the policy implemented in other jurisdictions worked to Australian actors' advantage, as the diffusion of the policy offered validation of the policy's efficacy. Various ideas proliferate in the literature as to why policy transfer occurs; constructivist diffusion theorists point to changes in ideas and the influence of global norms (e.g. Meyer et al. 1992), while coercion theorists point to power dynamics and changes in incentives (Owen 2002). In the transfer school, Dolowitz and Marsh (1996, 2000) point to reasons such as dissatisfaction among policy-makers or the public, perceived policy failures, or uncertainty. What we see in this case, however, is that transfer occurred in part due to a political decision to enable diffusion, in order to validate policy choices in both the 'exporter' and 'importer' jurisdictions. Where the transfer process is highly politicised, therefore, it could be inferred that this could speed up diffusion or transfer, as policy advocates seek to spread the idea as far as possible. Indeed, in this case, the very nature of the transfer process itself was determined in part by the need for policy-makers and NGOs to build relationships and coalitions in an effort to counteract transnational corporate actors' strategies in both the 'exporting' and 'importing' jurisdictions.

This volume has both provided new empirical data on the battle for standardised packaging in Europe and contributed new theoretical insights on the nature of policy transfer processes in multi-level polities. It has shown how the combination of complex, multi-level governance systems with networks of policy-makers and NGOs may give rise to policy transfer 'webs', potentially containing multiple consecutive and/or concurrent processes of both 'horizontal' and 'vertical' policy exchange. It has further demonstrated that a closer analytical look at the roles of transnational corporate actors is necessary within the policy transfer literature. We have demonstrated that TTCs not only sought to attack and disrupt transfer mechanisms that were facilitating the adoption of SP, but that they also developed their own 'counter-policy' transfer pathways. The impact on the success of the policy transfer process was mixed; while the TTCs achieved some success at the EU level, and induced a 'chilling effect' in some jurisdictions that delayed adopting the policy at the national level, in other ways the activities of the TTCs inadvertently encouraged the development of networks committed to the successful diffusion of the policy.

Bibliography

Baumgartner, F., & Jones, B. (1991). Agenda dynamics and policy subsystems. *The Journal of Politics, 53*(4), 1044–1074.

Benson, D., & Jordan, A. (2011). What have we learned from policy transfer research? Dolowitz and Marsh revisited. *Political Studies Review, 9*(3), 366–378.

Bomberg, E., & Peterson, J. (2000). *Policy transfer and Europeanization: Passing the Heineken Test?* (Queen's Papers on Europeanisation p0002). Queen's University Belfast.

Chapman, S., & Freeman, B. (2014). *Removing the emperor's clothes: Australia and tobacco plain packaging*. Sydney: Sydney University Press.

Costa, H., Gilmore, A. B., Peeters, S., McKee, M., & Stuckler, D. (2014). Quantifying the influence of the tobacco industry on EU governance: Automated content analysis of the EU Tobacco Products Directive. *Tobacco Control, 23*, 473–478.

Dobbin, F., Simmons, B., & Garrett, G. (2007). The global diffusion of public policies: Social construction, coercion, competition, or learning? *Annual Review of Sociology, 33*, 449–472.

Dolowitz, D. (2003). A policy-maker's guide to policy transfer. *The Political Quarterly, 74*(1), 101–108.

Dolowitz, D., & Marsh, D. (1996). Who learns what from whom: A review of the policy transfer literature. *Political Studies, 44*(2), 343–357.

Dolowitz, D., & Marsh, D. (2000). Learning from Abroad: The role of policy transfer in contemporary policy-making. *Governance, 13*(1), 5–23.

Dunlop, C. A. (2009). Policy transfer as learning: Capturing variation in what decision-makers learn from epistemic communities. *Policy Studies, 30*(3), 289–311.

Evans, M. (2009). Policy transfer in critical perspective. *Policy Studies, 30*(3), 243–268.

Evans, M., & Davies, J. (1999). Understanding policy transfer: A multi-level, multi-disciplinary perspective. *Public Administration, 77*(2), 361–385.

Gleditsch, K. S., & Ward, M. D. (2006). Diffusion and the spread of democratic institutions. *International Organisations, 60,* 911–933.

Hawkins, B., & Holden, C. (2016). A corporate veto on health policy? Global constitutionalism and investor-state dispute settlement. *Journal of Health Politics, Policy and Law, 13,* 1–19.

Hawkins, B., Holden, C., & Mackinder, S. (2018). A multi-level, multi-jurisdictional strategy: Transnational tobacco companies' attempts to obstruct tobacco packaging restrictions. *Global Public Health.* https://doi.org/10.1080/17441692.2018.1446997.

Holden, C., & Hawkins, B. (2017). Law, market building and public health in the European Union. *Global Social Policy,* 1–17.

Holden, C., & Lee, K. (2009). Corporate power and social policy: The political economy of the transnational tobacco companies. *Global Social Policy, 9*(3), 328–354.

Hudson, J., & Lowe, S. (2009). *Understanding the policy process: Analysing welfare policy and practice* (2nd ed.). Bristol: Policy Press.

Hurt, R. D., Ebbert, J. O., Muggli, M. E., Lockhart, N. J., & Robertson, C. R. (2009). Open doorway to truth: Legacy of the Minnesota tobacco trial. *Mayo Clinic Proceedings, 84*(5), 446–456.

Jarman, H. (2015). *The politics of trade and tobacco control.* Basingstoke: Palgrave Macmillan.

Jones, T., & Newburn, T. (2006). *Policy transfer and criminal justice.* Milton Keynes: Open University Press.

Jordan, A., Wurzel, R., Zito, A. R., & Brückner, L. (2003). European governance and the transfer of 'new' environmental policy instruments (NEPIs) in the European Union. *Public Administration, 81*(3), 555–574.

Kingdon, J. W. (1984). *Agendas, alternatives and public policies.* Boston, MA: Little, Brown.

MacKenzie, R., Mathers, A., Hawkins, B., Eckhardt, J., & Smith, J. (2018). The tobacco industry's challenge to standardised packaging: A comparative analysis of issue framing in public relations campaigns in four countries. *Health Policy, 122*(9), 1001–1011.

Meyer, J. W., Ramirez, F. O., & Soysal, Y. (1992). World expansion of mass education, 1870–1980. *Sociological Education, 65,* 128–149.

Owen, J. M. J. (2002). The foreign imposition of domestic institutions. *International Organizations, 56,* 375–409.

Peeters, S., Costa, H., Stuckler, D., McKee, M., & Gilmore, A. B. (2015). The revision of the 2014 European Tobacco Products Directive: An analysis of the

tobacco industry's attempts to 'break the health silo'. *Tobacco Control*. https://doi.org/10.1136/tobaccocontrol-2014-051919.
Pierson, C., & Castles, F. G. (2002). Australian antecedents of the Third Way. *Political Studies, 50*, 683–702.
Radaelli, C. (2000). Policy transfer in the European Union: Institutional isomorphism as a source of legitimacy. *Governance, 13*(1), 25–43.
Savell, E., Gilmore, A. B., Fooks, G., & Derrick, G. E. (2014). How does the tobacco industry attempt to influence marketing regulations? A systematic review. *PLoS One, 9*, e87389. https://doi.org/10.1371/journal.pone.0087389.
Smith, K. E., Savell, E., & Gilmore, A. B. (2013). What is known about tobacco industry efforts to influence tobacco tax? A systematic review of empirical studies. *Tobacco Control, 22*(2), 144–153.
Stone, D. (2004). Transfer agents and global networks in the 'transnationalization' of policy. *Journal of European Public Policy, 11*(3), 545–566.
Stone, D. (2012). Transfer and translation of policy. *Policy Studies, 33*(6), 483–499.
World Health Organization (WHO). (2003). *WHO framework convention on tobacco control* [Online]. Available at https://www.who.int/tobacco/framework/WHO_FCTC_english.pdf. Accessed 5 February 2019.

Index

B. Hawkins et al., *The Battle for Standardised Cigarette Packaging in Europe*, Palgrave Studies in Public Health Policy Research,
https://doi.org/10.1007/978-3-030-31034-9

9783030310332